Geriatric Medicine and Gerontology

Edited by Edward T. Zawada Jr.

Published in London, United Kingdom

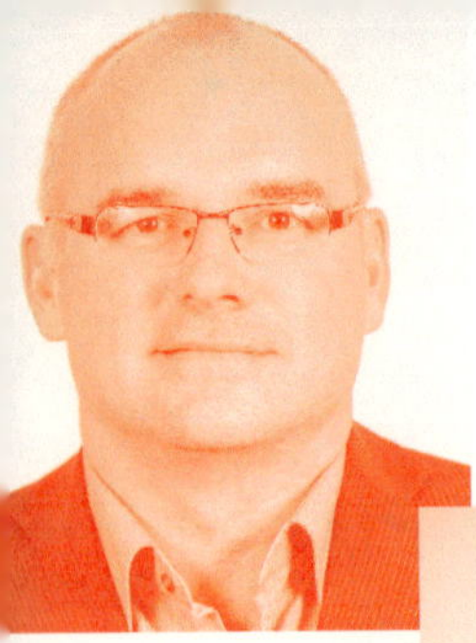
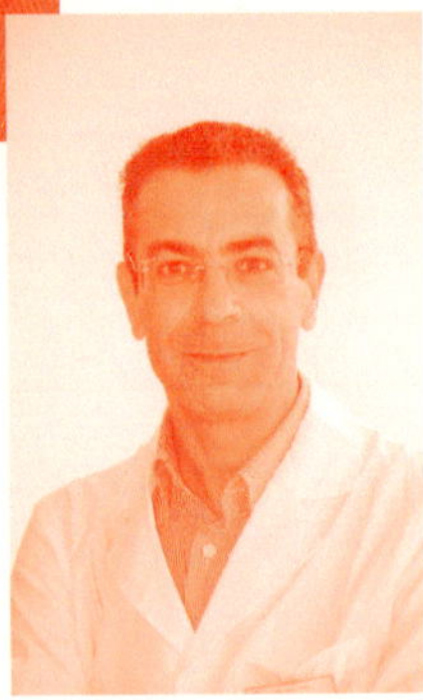
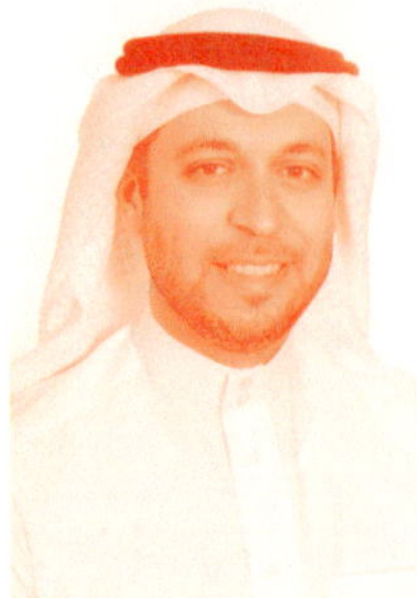
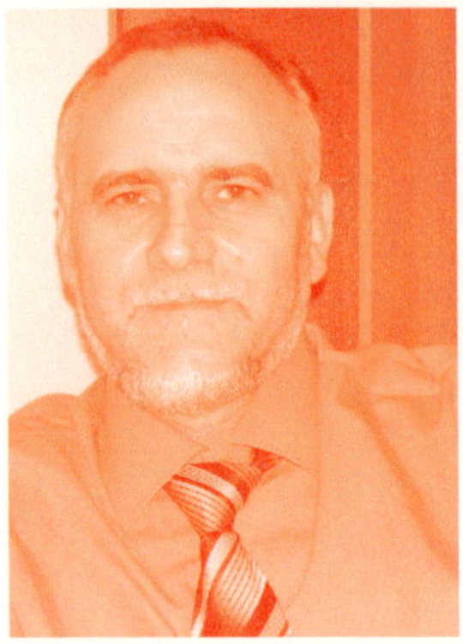
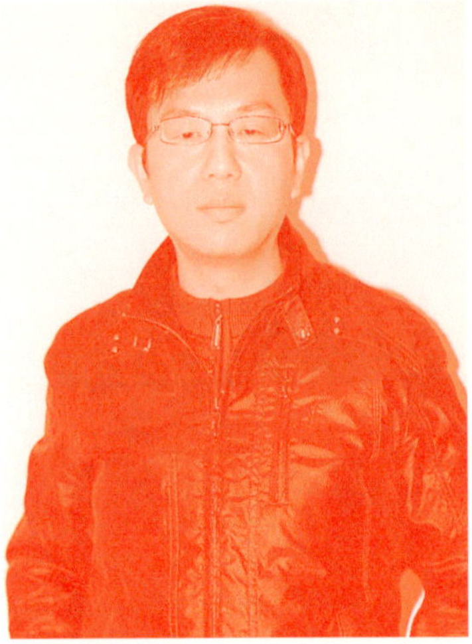
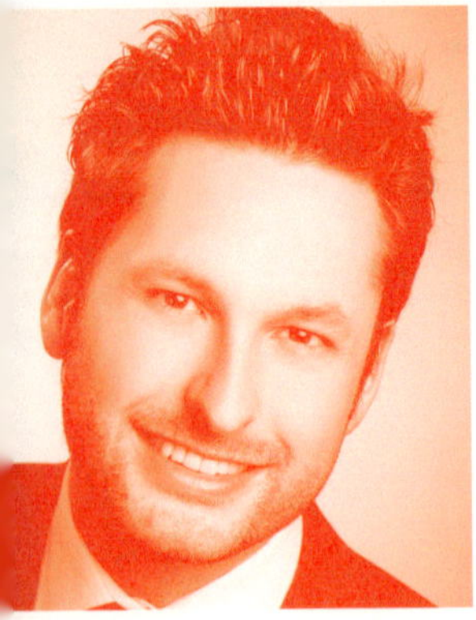
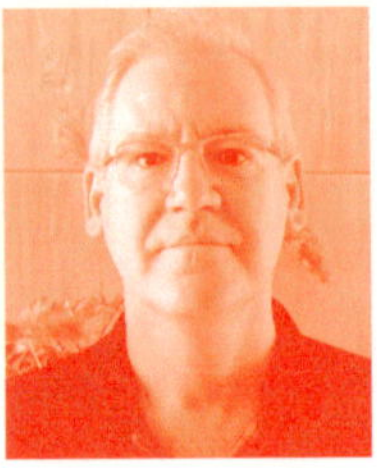

IntechOpen

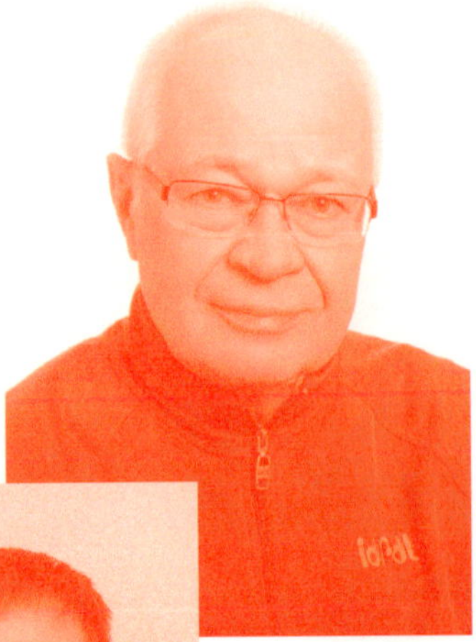
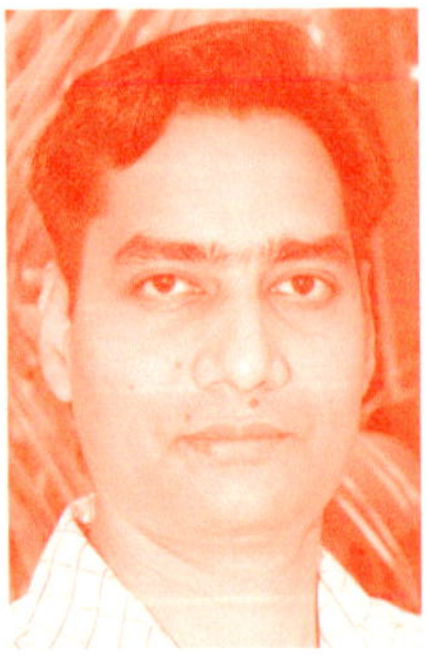
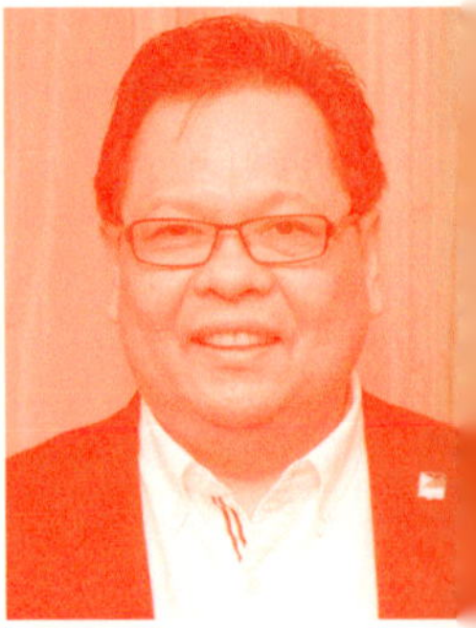
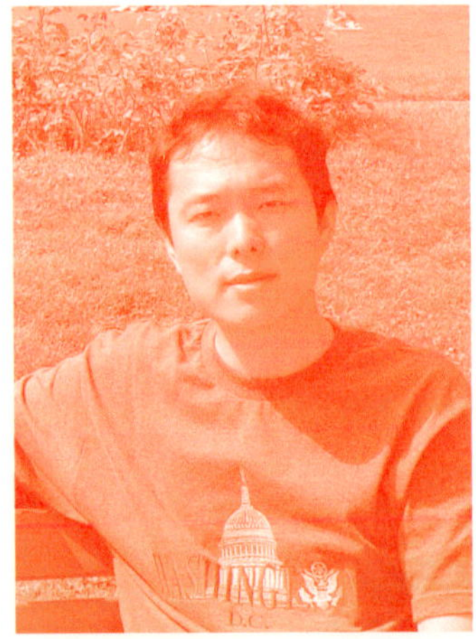
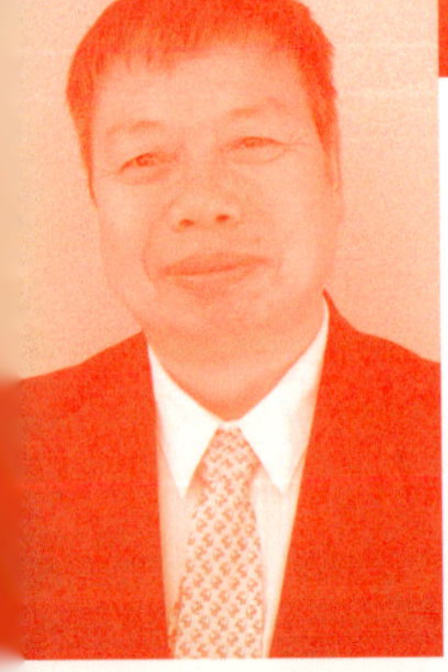
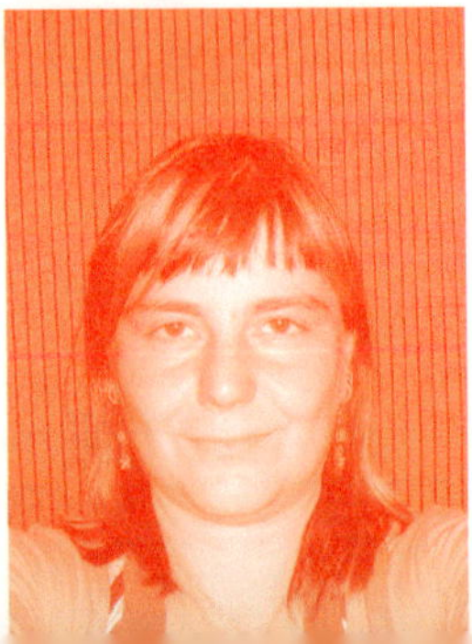

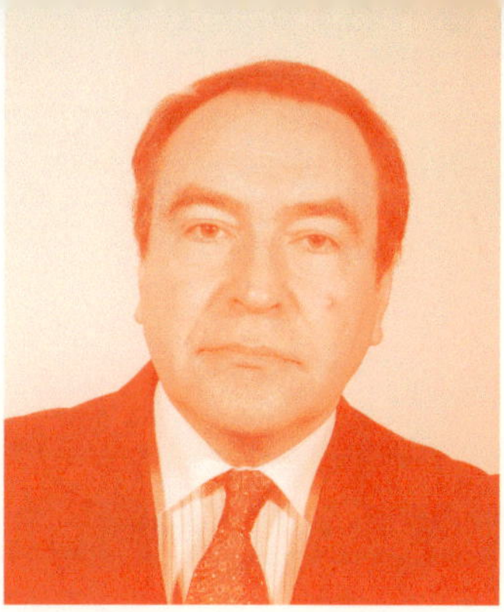
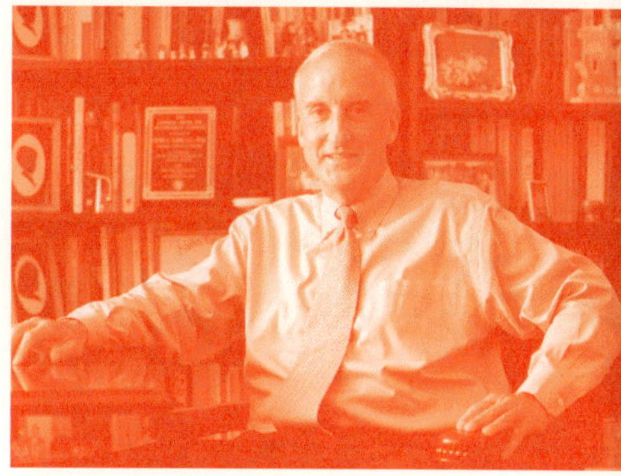
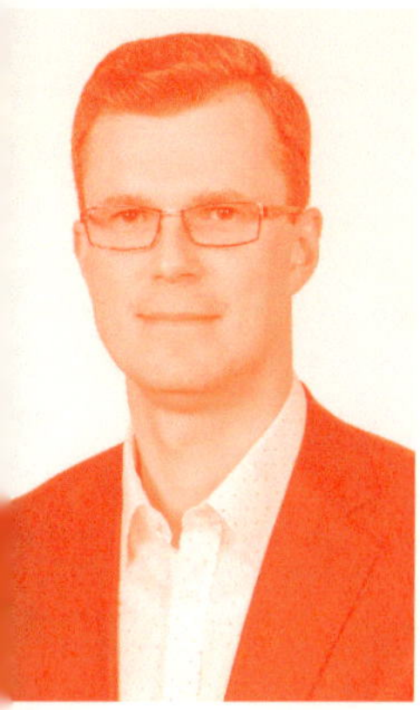
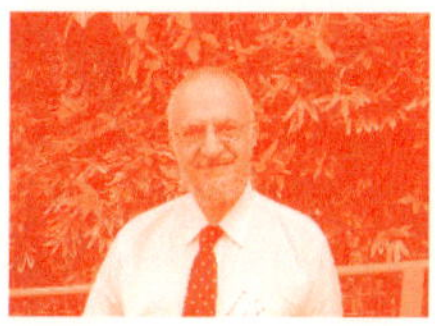
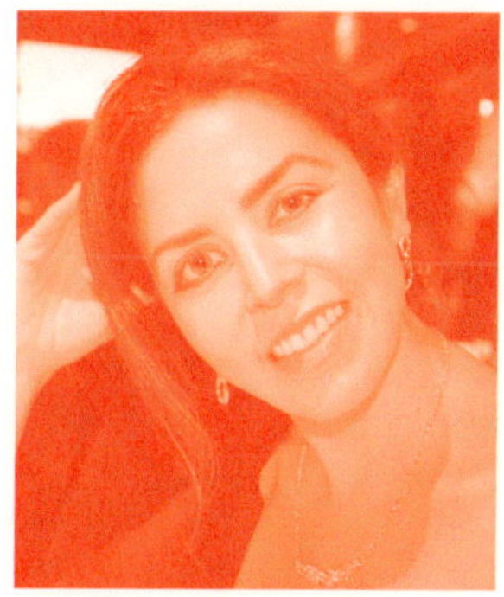

Supporting open minds since 2005

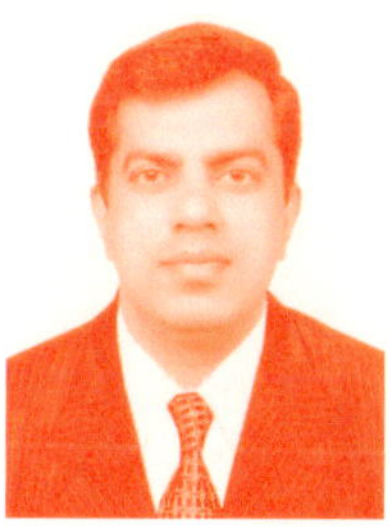
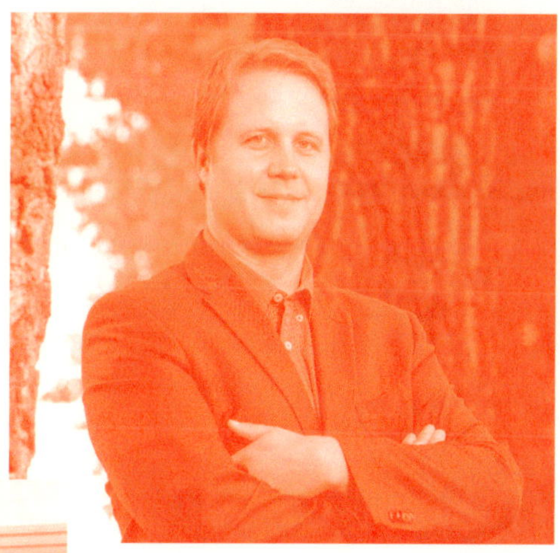
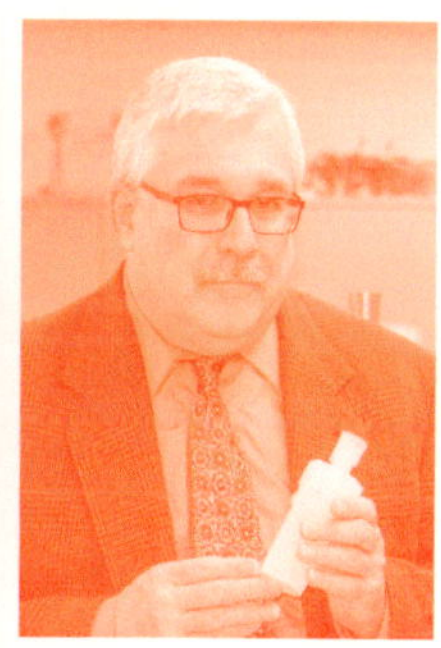
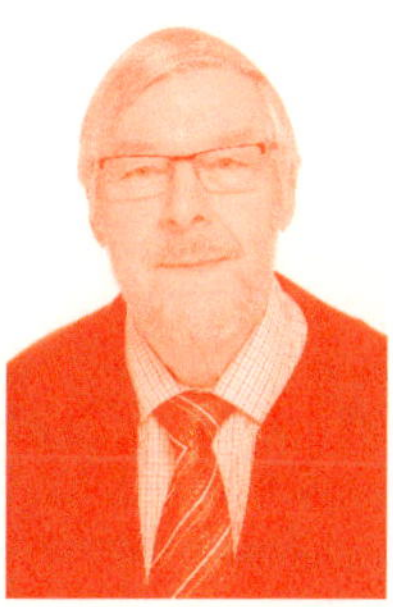
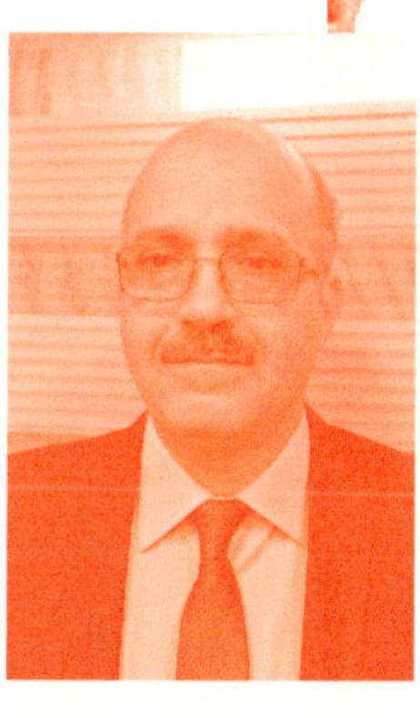
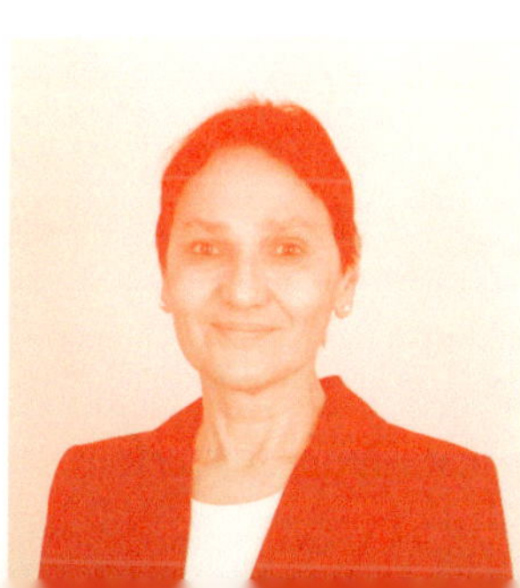
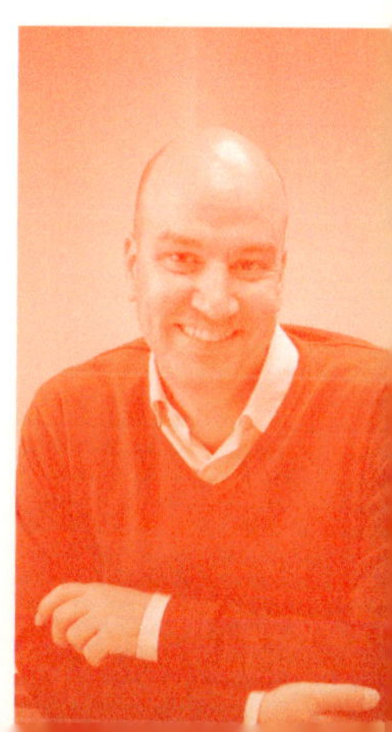

Geriatric Medicine and Gerontology
http://dx.doi.org/10.5772/intechopen.77654
Edited by Edward T. Zawada Jr.

Contributors
Marcos Eduardo Scheicher, Natália Moya Rodrigues Pereira, Francesca Romana Greco, Davide Seripa, Monica Greco, Grazia D'Onofrio, Daniele Sancarlo, Filomena Ciccone, Antonio Mangiacotti, Demet Özbabalık Adapınar, Ahmet Onur Keskin, Nazlı Durmaz, Gülgün Uncu, Ebru Erzurumluoglu, Zerrin Yıldırım, Nese Tuncer, Meritxell Espino-Guarch, Moza Al-Kowari, Martha Alvarado Ibarra, José Antonio De la Peña Celaya, Cláudia Tiemi Mituuti, Giédre Berretin-Felix, Marcela Maria Alves da Silva, Iracema Leroi, Sabina Vatter, Emmanuel Andrès, Laurent Meyer, Abrar-Ahmad Zulfiqar, Mohamed Hajjam, Samy Talha, Sylvie Ervé, Jawad Hajjam, Nathalie Jeandidier, Amir Hajjam El Hassani, Ettore Bergamini, Gabriella Cavallini, Edward T. Zawada Jr.

First published in London, United Kingdom, 2019 by IntechOpen
IntechOpen is the global imprint of INTECHOPEN LIMITED, registered in England and Wales, registration number: 11086078, 7th floor, 10 Lower Thames Street, London, EC3R 6AF, United Kingdom
Printed in Croatia

British Library Cataloguing-in-Publication Data
A catalogue record for this book is available from the British Library

Additional hard and PDF copies can be obtained from orders@intechopen.com

Geriatric Medicine and Gerontology
Edited by Edward T. Zawada Jr.
p. cm.
Print ISBN 978-1-78984-389-7
Online ISBN 978-1-78984-390-3
eBook (PDF) ISBN 978-1-78984-144-2

For EU product safety concerns:
IN TECH d.o.o., Prolaz Marije Krucifikse Kozulić 3, 51000 Rijeka, Croatia, info@intechopen.com or visit our website at intechopen.com.

Meet the editor

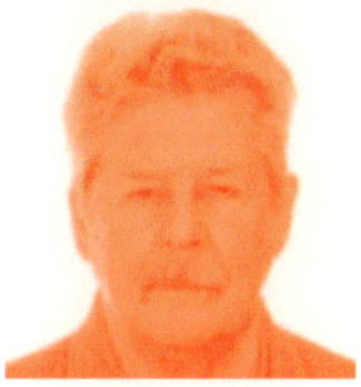

Edward T. Zawada Jr. graduated summa cum laude from Loyola University in 1969 and summa cum laude from Loyola-Stritch School of Medicine in 1973. He trained at the University of California at Los Angeles (UCLA) from 1973 to 1978. His faculty positions include UCLA, University of Utah, Medical College of Virginia, and University of South Dakota. Other positions include professor and chairman emeritus, Department of Internal Medicine, University of South Dakota, Sanford School of Medicine; and Bush Foundation of Minnesota Sabbatical Fellowship in Critical Care, Department of Anesthesiology at the University of Iowa in 2009. Dr. Zawada Jr. is board certified by the American Board of Internal Medicine in Internal Medicine, Nephrology, Geriatrics, and Critical Care Medicine. Other board certifications include Nutrition and Clinical Pharmacology. He is a Master of the American College of Physicians and Fellow of the American College of Critical Care Medicine, the American Society of Nephrology, the American Society of Hypertension, the American College of Chest Physicians, the American College of Clinical Pharmacology, the American College of Nutrition, and the American Heart Association.

Contents

Preface

The science of changes in metabolism, gene expression, tissue function, and organ physiology as humans age has been expanding exponentially since the 1980s when a clinical specialty was created by the American Boards of Internal Medicine and Family Medicine. Although often used interchangeably, gerontology is considered to stress the psychological, functional, and social problems facing elders, while geriatrics is considered to focus on the physiologic, metabolic, tissue, and organ processes that result in medical problems. Both fields are concerned with quality of life as individuals reach the decades of life between 60 years of age and death.

This volume is a collection of reports organized into three sections. The first section is an introduction to the evolution of knowledge considered to be inclusive in the clinical specialty of geriatrics. It also includes an example of an important area of gerontology, that of identity changes in the aging woman. The second section is devoted to cutting-edge issues in diagnosing and managing dementia. This is the largest section in this book and concludes with a chapter on the future treatment of Alzheimer's disease. Finally, a third section deals with newer developments in geriatrics and covers hearing loss and acute and chronic lymphoproliferative diseases. The section concludes with a very important chapter on the use of electrical stimulation of nerves and muscles to reduce morbidity in a variety of neurologic degenerative diseases that occur in the elderly.

I have been involved in the care of the elderly for more than forty-five years. The chapters in this book present a short survey of the transformation of the field that has occurred over this time. I thank all the contributors who give this book a worldwide perspective. All reports dealing with elders and their medical, psychological, and social problems are more important than ever as we are in the middle of the wave of baby boomers who have passed the age of 60 years.

Edward T. Zawada Jr.
University of South Dakota,
United States of America

Section 1

Geriatrics as a Specialty

Chapter 1

Introductory Chapter: Geriatrics

Edward T. Zawada

1. Introduction

Geriatrics has been identified as a subspecialty by virtue of a board certification since the mid-1980s by the American Board of Internal Medicine. The original core of knowledge was primarily the extension of the diagnoses and management of diseases of organ systems to the three age groups over the age of 60 years: young-old was 60–70, old was 70–80, and old-old was over 80 years of age. At that time I became interested in geriatrics by focusing on elders with renal and urology diseases [1]. At the beginning I researched the anatomic and physiologic changes of the kidney and urinary system, and then later each other major organ system of the body. My work in renal and urologic diseases led to editing my first book in the field [2]. As I delved into caring for the elderly, I became exposed to the knowledge of problems which are outside of the individual organ systems like "falls" or problems which affect every organ system like "geropharmacology." Over the decades since then, the role of the geriatrician who is the primary care provider for the elderly requires knowledge in a multitude of other specialties beyond internal medicine such as ophthalmology, ENT, audiology, neurology, orthopedics, and physiatry. I will present the earliest skills needed for the care of the elderly followed by the newest skills now incorporated into the subject matter of geriatrics. The chapters in this book mostly represent a catalog of the newer skills.

2. Previous geriatric skills

2.1 Geriatric assessment

One of the first skills I learned when preparing for practice in geriatrics was that of geriatric assessment. I saw the amazing statistics of increased diagnostic accuracy, prevention of iatrogenic problems, and improved functional status which translated to better quality of life. We developed this tool for our practice [1] and spent the next 2 years unraveling difficult diagnostic and management problems for the patients in our clinic. Our multidisciplinary team included a nurse, physician, pharm. D., social worker, mental health expert, physical therapist, occupational therapist, dietician, and speech therapist. Our day consisted of intake by the nurse, exam by the physician, sequential evaluation by each of the other team members, and contact by the physician to the patient's referring physician. After a preliminary meeting of the team, the patient and family were invited to a brainstorming session in which the findings were reviewed and additional questions were invited. Then a second team meeting finalized our findings and recommendations which were again presented to the family and patient and transmitted to the referring physician. I realized that the complex problems of the elderly with their age-related lack of compensation ability, their multiple comorbid conditions, and the large number of socioeconomic issues that influenced the quality of life of these patients could only be completely dealt with by this tremendous manpower commitment. We literally committed 1 full day per patient.

2.2 Nutrition

I had a prior background in nutritional research and was board-certified by the American College of Nutrition (now absorbed into the American Society of Parenteral and Enteral Nutrition or ASPET). In light of the huge number of patients whose medical and socioeconomic problems and limited resources led to nutritional deficiencies, we undertook a project to provide supplements to elders involved in communal meal programs like Meals on Wheels or congregate dining at senior centers [2]. We called the program as our "Meal Mate" program.

2.3 Pharmacology

We discovered the problem of polypharmacy in many of our clinic patients. We sought not only to streamline their medications but to reach out to our rural community as well [3]. We would bring our team to community centers after announcing free consultation for medication simplification, and we offered education concerning possible adverse reactions and adverse drug interactions. The recommendations were made after consulting with their primary care providers. A written summary of recommendations was given to the patients and transmitted to their primary physicians. We were among the earliest to use the term "MedRed" program.

2.4 Nephrology

I became interested in geriatrics when I decided to focus my primary specialty of nephrology to the care of elders with renal insufficiency. My collaborators and I put together what in my opinion was the first subspecialty textbook of geriatrics [4]. My basic research team and I focused on factors which led to age-related changes in renal anatomy and physiology independent of diseases [5]. We explored the dietary and other means to slow down such aging of the kidneys.

3. Current skills

The American Geriatrics Society has published its syllabus to serve as a compendium of the core information considered as the standard data base for geriatricians to be able to successfully care for their patients in modern day practice [6]. As mentioned above, besides the "internal medicine" organ system diseases, there are large sections devoted to visual loss, hearing loss, syncope, dizziness, falls, frailty, swallowing problems, nutrition management, pressure wounds, behavior disturbances, delusions, dermatology, addiction, and gynecology.

In addition, the current practice of geriatrics requires an incredible knowledge of socioeconomic management issues such as ethics and advanced directives, elder abuse, insurance coverage and payments, mobility, and driving competence.

4. Conclusions

In conclusion, the field of geriatrics has undergone a transformation from the hospital-based application of internal medicine subspecialty care to the outpatient broader application of multiple medical specialties as deliverable by office practice.

From a solitary or episodic intervention, it has expanded to a continuous, ongoing set of interventions designed not so much to perform diagnostic studies or prescribe curative medications, but instead to improve mobility, mentation, and special senses and in that way improve quality of life.

Author details

Edward T. Zawada
Department of Internal Medicine, Sanford School of Medicine, University of South Dakota, South Dakota, United States

*Address all correspondence to: ezawada@sio.midco.net

References

[1] Schrader S, Blue R, Zawada E Jr, Millder D, Jensen G, Hill P, et al. Strengthening geriatric knowledge and use of interdisciplinary teams among allied health students and practitioners. Educational Gerontology: An International Journal. 1999;**25**(1):51-56

[2] Schrader SI, Schrank M, Blue R, Zawada ET Jr, Trujillo AI, Alavi FK. Meal mate: Improving the nutritional status of elders using a mild-based nutritional supplement. South Dakota Journal of Medicine. 1995;**48**:301-311

[3] Schrader SI, Dressing B, Zawada ET Jr, Blue R. The medication reduction (MEDRED) project. Combating polypharmacy in South Dakota elders through community-based interventions. South Dakota Journal of Medicine. 1996;**49**(12):441-448

[4] Zawada ET Jr, Sica DA, editors. Geriatric Nephrology and Urology. Littleton Massachusetts: Wright PSG; 1985. 558 p. Library of Congress Catalog card number 84-18927

[5] Zawada ET Jr. The aging kidney. In: Massry S, Glassock R, editors. Textbook of Nephrology. 2nd ed. Baltimore MD: Williams and Wilkins; 1989. pp. 996-1002

[6] Medina-Walpole A, Pacala JT, Potter JE. Geriatric Review Syllabus. New York: American Geriatrics Society Publishers; 2016. Library of Congress Control Number 2016931643

Chapter 2

Old Age and Women's Identity

Greco Francesca Romana, D'Onofrio Grazia, Seripa Davide, Ciccone Filomena, Sancarlo Daniele, Mangiacotti Antonio and Greco Monica

Abstract

Female identity is a dynamic concept, and it has been a very discussed issue by contemporary cultural critic. How does old age affect identity construction and perception in elderly woman? Has feminine gender an impact in subjective well-being? Psychological changes of midlife women have been as conflicting as the idea that society has about them. Personality changes after young adulthood in women is a controversial matter. Erikson proposed that women might not develop identities in early adulthood as men do. In fact, he argued that women develop them later, in the context of an intimate relationship. Moreover, identity development appears to have important consequences for midlife well-being. For example, Vandewater et al. found that women's midlife well-being was facilitated by earlier attainment of a well-articulated identity. In these situations accomplishment of developmentally earlier tasks (identity formation) sets the stage for later psychological health. Our work sheds additional light on how women live this period of life in terms of happiness and purpose of life.

Keywords: old age, identity, woman, well-being

1. Introduction

Aging is a complex and natural process both for women and men, but there are some differences about the way they become confident with it. In fact, in women, the representation of emotional and cognitive feeling concerning identity is very different than in men [1].

It has been widely assumed that women of middle age usher in a long period of decline toward death and that therefore it will be associated with an increase in thoughts about death and mortality, as well as with declines in perceived physical, relational, and psychological capacities [2].

As Gergen highlighted women have always been associated to their reproductive capacities. Therefore, aging may have a great impact on women's self-identity as it can be interpreted as a loss of power [3].

However, there is an evidence that some aspects of women's well-being (positive relations with others and personal growth) are somewhat better than men's at all ages and none are worse [4].

Moreover, Montepare in 1996 found that middle-aged women had more favorable body images, in some respects, than younger women.

Finally, it is generally assumed that concern about aging, especially the physical processes associated with it, is more common and age-appropriate among the elderly than the middle-aged [5].

Since the turn of the century, there has been enormous progress in aging research in many fields.

In this book chapter, we focused on women and their identity.

The aim of this chapter is to shed additional light on women's identity and how they live their "silver years" in terms of happiness and purpose of life.

Finally, our work shows how aging depends on women's mental attitude, not only on physical changes related to biological age.

2. Emotional aging and women's well-being

In contrast to decline associated with physical and cognitive aging, emotional aging appears to improve with age.

Furthermore, dispositional tendencies, life events, and individuals' management of such events can all influence whether well-being improves or deteriorates with age.

Nevertheless, researches carry out that reasonably high levels of affective well-being and emotional stability are normal at least until after adults reach 70 or 80 years of age [6].

Experts proposed many theories about emotional aging.

Some theories on life-span emotional-motivational development highlight that normative shifts in emotional goals and strategies in adulthood are common in women's and men's adulthood. On the other hand, socio-emotional selectivity theory focuses on the importance of the acceptance of life-end in order to experience pleasant moment at present. This would help people to focus on present challenges rather than eluding them aiming to future rewards. Getting old is physiologically linked to the concept of endings; therefore, the theory predicts motivational changes during aging. This concept may be valid also for those people with a short life expectancy [7].

Dynamic integration theory underlines that as aging is linked to cognitive ability decrease, elderly often have problems with social integration and make great efforts when experiencing negative feelings [8].

The life-span theory of control holds that individuals' capacity to control their environment and achieve their developmental goals declines in older adulthood [9].

Consequently, when experiencing a new condition, elderly tend to change the self rather to the situation itself. On the other hand, authors suggest that experiencing and practicing emotional situations may play a positive role on elderly ability of managing them [10, 11].

In conclusion, according to the model of selection, optimization, and compensation, the ability of shifting between emotional preferences helps elderly to contrast progressive cognitive decline. As explained by Howden and Meyer structural and anatomical changes occurring during aging have a great impact of the concept of well-being. They noticed that structural degradation and functional slowing of the autonomic system may diminish physiological arousal after exposure to emotional stimuli, thereby reducing the impact of negative events.

However, once an autonomic reaction starts, the same mechanism can lengthen physiological reactions, thereby increasing the duration of negative emotional states [12, 13].

3. Women's experiences of body image and their identity in aging

Highlighting the complexities of women's psychological and physical aspects of aging, clinical psychology suggests that women over 50 currently cover over 17.2% of the total population and this percentage is expected to increase [14].

DOI: http://dx.doi.org/10.5772/intechopen.84740

Of concern, over the last decade, we have observed an increase in the number of middle-aged and older women presenting for inpatient eating disorder treatment and a rise in the prevalence of obesity in women aged over 60 years [15, 16].

However, our understanding of women's experiences of body image in relation to the aging process is limited.

To date, most of the body image research has been on younger samples and has focused on satisfaction with weight and size [17].

A focused research on middle-aged and old women's concept of their body is necessary in order to target researchers' attention. With this aim the Gender and Body Image study was developed [18].

This study was conducted to capture the thoughts, feelings, and attitudes that women at middle age have about their bodies and the experience of aging.

This research gathered survey-based information related to body image, health, identity, and aging from 1,849 women over age 50 across the United States.

Quantitative data revealed body dissatisfaction, eating disorder symptoms, and extreme weight control methods in a significant number of these women.

According to other studies, it was also demonstrated that body dissatisfaction in women appears to be fairly stable across age despite the fact that body appreciation increases [19].

It is commonly known that aging is associated with unwelcome changes in physical appearance, increased dependency on others, and negative societal stereotypes [20].

Thus, middle and old age are generally seen as a period of decline in Western society, a problem with particular relevance for women due to Western society's long history of placing value on physical appearance, youth, and thinness [21–23].

To date, several interview-based qualitative studies illustrate the contradictory nature of women's experiences of aging and body image [24]. While aging women experience unwelcome changes in physical appearance. At the same time, they become more focused on physical health and more rejecting about social pressures related to appearance [25].

Unfortunately, all these qualitative studies refer to interviews conducted on narrow age groups or focused on one particular aspect of aging (e.g., weight and body size).

The GABI analysis, however, inquired on perceptions and experiences of women over 50 focusing on body image, aging, and identity in order to generate ideas for future study and to inform clinical practice.

Women enrolled in this study were interested both in physical and psychological aspects of aging.

This topic was identified in another qualitative study of aging and body image among older women in a narrower age group [24] and supports quantitative research indicating that body image becomes more complex with age.

According to similar researches [26, 27], women were disappointed to weight and metabolism change, which were considered as signs of aging.

Many of the enrolled female subjects referred that as experiencing body changes, cognitive adaptations to the physical experience of aging and the psychological experience of body image simultaneously changed. Women referred that unforeseen body change acceptance was a frightening task; on this matter menopause was described as a crucial period as women referred contrasting feelings. They have to face the occurrence of physical changes due to their old age, regretting their younger bodies. Older women strongly voiced a sense of injustice in their aging experience, recounting external pressures from the society about appearance that were different for aging men.

Women interviewed in this study described an awareness of these internal shifts, acknowledging that they were less interested in adhering to the societal expectations, yet still felt challenged to adhere to them regardless of age [28].

Women commented on feelings of invisibility and irrelevance, a phenomenon that has also been highlighted [29].

The lack of representation of aging women in the media documented in quantitative reports did not go unnoticed by our participants [30].

Women commented on the increasing importance of self-care, noting that caring for their physical health assumed priority over physical appearance as they grew older, concurring with previous descriptions [23, 31].

Young women's confidence is usually based on beauty and appearance. On the other hand, old women consider health and physical autonomy as the most relevant values. However, society does not seem to accord to these changes.

In fact women reported to be undervalued while getting old. As Twigg and Majima remark, women aim to be still considered for their capacities, and although their priorities may shift toward functionality, they are still interested on their appearance. In fact they still enjoy clothing and cosmetic shopping [32].

Women asserted that although their priorities may shift toward functionality, this does not mean that appearance no longer matters.

4. When the old age become a challenge

Being old can be a challenge. Senses become less sophisticated, friends are fewer, and stress easily increases. Additionally, loneliness, sense of dependence from others, anxiety, sadness, and apathy are some of the most common feelings and emotions perceived by the older.

How to escape from that? Many therapeutic interventions were proposed, especially for women:

4.1 Dance therapy

Dance therapy for the elderly is a cognitive and social activity which improves levels of resilience and adaptation to the stresses of aging [33]. Working both on physical and intellectual aspects, dance sessions showed great results concerning self-esteem, communication, and general well-being.

4.2 Pet-assisted therapy to the health of the elderly

Recently, there has been a growing interest toward elderly's affective and emotional needs.

The aim of relational therapies is to increase the understanding of those needs and patients' well-being.

As well as being wonderful companions, studies revealed that pets provide significant health benefits to their owner [34]. Many studies were also conducted on ill subjects. As Sollami et al. underlined, pet therapy could have a great emotional and social impact, bringing relief to patients and their family members but also to health professionals [35].

5. The incredible art of gossip: An healthy women habit

Gossip is an healthy women habit. Getting older people have to face up new and unpleasant situations, and social contact plays a key role on the ability to overcome them.

Once again, men and women react differently, using various cognitive and social strategies. During aging many cognitive functions (i.e., memory) may decrease and deafness occurs; however, women keep on being curious about neighbors' and friends' news. Gossip is more than an ordinary behavior. In fact, the Konstanz Department of Psychology in Germany has recently pointed out the importance of communication as the heart of social and cultural life [36]. Being capable of building relationships represents a powerful ability that guides human and social intelligence over the entire life span.

Hartung and Renner underline the central role of relationships. They suggest that social curiosity and the tendency to gossip are inherently related to each other. In fact they represent two different social functioning drives. On the one hand, curiosity is described as the main component for development and learning behaviors. The main curiosity functions are creating interpersonal strings and facilitating the feeling of belonging to others. People with interpersonal curiosity are more sociable and resilient to stressful events. Therefore, they need to control social world in order to feel safe and relaxed. To sum up, curiosity is defined as the "drive to know."

On the other hand, gossip is generally described as "an entertainment of pleasure."

Information, friendship, influence, and entertainment are considered to be the main social functions. Sharing gossip and news stands as a dynamic strategy in order to socialize, create relationship, and prevent from outsiders' exclusion.

Gossip represents a type of exploratory and learning behavior in a word that is going to be more complex, especially for elderly people.

6. It is time to get online: the importance of being in touch and the role of social media

To date, social media and technology play a central role in our social life, and they are considered to be the best and easiest ways to communicate as they allow people to keep in touch with friends reducing distance. It is interesting to consider how is elderly approach to 2.0 reality and how it could have a crucial role in their daily life. Discussion boards, social networks, blogs, videos, and virtual reality are all ways to share information, bringing people together and improving social contact, and they can prevent elderly from social isolation.

Denecke et al. suggest that the "social media phenomenon" is increasing through the elderly, especially through those who suffer from chronic illness [37].

Moreover, peer-to-peer healthcare is emerging as a source of information and social support for chronically ill patients.

Nowadays, technology and social media represent a great opportunity to support and prevent social isolation. The last one is the major seniors' noxious factors. Social media also stand as a place to share information and personal stories. This virtual place could be a chance to create a fertile and stimulating open space in order to share interpersonal feelings and fears.

Virtual reality is another way elderly could use to express themselves. Arlati et al. conducted an interesting research on this matter. The aim of the study was to improve the patient's adherence to treatments, promoting collaboration and competition using virtual reality.

Researchers proposed a dual-task training program. They asked users to cycle on an uncommon bike while recognizing target animals as they appear along the way. The chance of training with other users in order to reduce the risk of social isolation was also given. Using "social bike," users can choose the multiplayer mode, in order to stimulate competition or cooperation with the others [38].

7. Conclusions

Before a woman becomes old, a long journey has just begun from the adolescents to juvenile period and from adult to old age.

Usually, the old age is commonly viewed as a sort of the final destination instead of the start of something knew.

As long-term memory appears to be reinforced by the time, also identity seems to be more stable and temperament, and character is already intrinsically connected to each other.

Old age is considered as a fully formed stone where the heart and mind are strictly connected.

Despite off, many authors suggest that before women become old, she could start to have some typical deficit as amnestic and neurocognitive problem, going through the mild cognitive impairment.

This is a critical stage in which the couple begins to decline, when they deal with losses, support the middle generation, and conduct a life review.

In this stage, usually considered between 65 years old, men and especially women are more sensitive to adverse events and health problem and begin to be more frailty.

Frailty is an important factor in functional and cognitive emotional decline, morbidity, and mortality for some older people.

Actually, anxiety, and depressive symptoms are much common in elderly people especially in women.

In older age, loneliness, social isolation, feeling of contribution/uselessness, lack of leisure activities, anxiety for the health, social deprivation, and depression are increasing [39].

In 2015, a writer and illustrator Matthew Johnstone tells the story of overcoming the "black dog of depression" [40].

He presents depression as a black dog, and it is clear to explain how depression is largely preventable and treatable.

The black dog could reduce the ability of concentrating, doing everything you were used to appreciate before, fear of being with other people, and constantly having fear to be discovered by other people's exhausting energy.

It could make you sad until damaging your identity.

Getting old with good attitudes like managing stressful events with resilience and being compassionate with other people could be a strategy to live better.

When a woman gets old, the frailty of identity and personality increase, and this is the reason why prevention is important to do not present these symptoms.

Being resilient, having a good relation with other people, and conducting a sport exercise are demonstrated to be essential on mental health overcoming the black dog [40].

In conclusion, our work shows how aging depends on women's mental attitude, not only on physical changes related to biological age [41].

Author details

Greco Francesca Romana*, D'Onofrio Grazia, Seripa Davide, Ciccone Filomena, Sancarlo Daniele, Mangiacotti Antonio and Greco Monica
Geriatric Unit, Department of Medical Sciences, IRCCS Casa Sollievo della Sofferenza, San Giovanni Rotondo, Italy

*Address all correspondence to: fra.greco93@gmail.com

References

[1] Vandewater EA, Ostrove JM, Stewart AJ. Predicting women's well-being in midlife: The importance of personality development and social role involvements. Journal of Personality and Social Psychology. 1997;**72**(5):1147-1160

[2] Stewart AJ, Ostrove JM, Helson R. Middle aging in women: Patterns of personality change from the 30s to the 50s. Journal of Adult Development. 2001;**8**(1):23-37

[3] Gergen MM. Finished at 40: Women's development within the patriarchy. Psychology of Women Quarterly. 1990;**14**:471-494

[4] Ryff CD, Singer B. Psychological well-being: Meaning, measurement, and implications for psychotherapy research. Psychotherapy and Psychosomatics. 1996;**65**:14-23

[5] Montepare JM. Actual and subjective age-related differences in women's attitudes toward their bodies across the lifespan. Journal of Adult Development. 1996;**3**:171-182

[6] Teachman BA. Aging and negative affect: The rise and fall and rise of anxiety and depression symptoms. Psychology and Aging. 2006;**21**(1):201-207

[7] Fung HH, Carstensen LL, Lutz AM. Influence of time on social preferences: Implications for life-span development. Psychology and Aging. 1999;**14**:595-604

[8] Vief G et al. Dynamic integration: Affect, cognition, and the self in adulthood. Current Directions in Psychological Science. 2003;**12**:201-206

[9] Heckhausen J, Schulz R. A life-span theory of control. Psychological Review. 1995;**102**:284-304

[10] Fields F. Everyday problem solving and emotion: An adult developmental perspective. Current Directions in Psychological Science. 2007;**16**:26-31

[11] Scheibe S, Blanchard-Fields F. Effects of regulating emotions on cognitive performance: What is costly for young adults is not so costly for older adults. Psychology and Aging. 2009;**24**:217-223

[12] Cacioppo JT, Berntson GG, Klein DJ, Poehlmann KM. Psychophysiology of emotion across the life span. In: Schaie KW, Lawton MP, editors. Annual Review of Gerontology and Geriatrics. Vol. 17: Focus on emotion and adult development. New York: Springer; 1998. pp. 27-74

[13] Charles ST, Piazza JR, Luong G, Almeida DA. Now you see it, now you don't: Age differences in affective reactivity to social tensions. Psychology and Aging. 2009;**24**:645-653

[14] Howden LM, Meyer JA. Age and Sex Composition. 2010 Census Briefs. 2010. Retrieved May 2011, 2011

[15] Ackard DM, Richter S, Frisch MJ, Mangham D, Cronemeyer CL. Eating disorder treatment among women forty and older: Increases in prevalence over time and comparisons to young adult patients. Journal of Psychosomatic Research. 2013;**74**(2):175-178. DOI: 10.1016/j.jpsychores.2012.10.014. PubMed: 23332534

[16] Pike KM, Dunne PE, Addai E. Expanding the boundaries: Reconfiguring the demographics of the "typical" eating disordered patient. Current Psychiatry Reports. 2013;**15**(11):411. DOI: 10.1007/s11920-013-0411-2. PubMed: 24122512

[17] Grogan S. Body image and health contemporary perspectives. Journal of

Health Psychology. 2006;**11**(4):523-530. PubMed: 16769732

[18] Hofmeier SM, Runfola CD, Sala M, Gagne DA, Brownley KA, Bulik CM. Body image, aging, and identity in women over 50: The gender and body image (GABI) study. Journal of Women and Aging. 2017; **29**(1):3-14. DOI: 10.1080/08952841.2015.1065140

[19] Öberg P, Tornstam L. Body images among men and women of different ages. Ageing and Society. 1999;**19**(05):629-644

[20] Nettleton S, Watson J. The Body in Everyday Life. Routledge. Psychology Press; 1998

[21] Furman F. Facing the Mirror: Older Women and Beauty Shop Culture. Routledge; 2013

[22] Laws G. Understanding Ageism: Lessons from Feminism and Postmodernism. The Gerontologist. 1995;**35**(1):112-118

[23] Twigg J. The body, gender, and age: Feminist insights in social gerontology. Journal of Aging Studies. 2004;**18**(1): 59-73. PubMed: 7890196

[24] Liechty T. Yes, I worry about my weight... but for the most part I'm content with my body: Older women's body dissatisfaction alongside contentment. Journal of Women and Aging. 2012;**24**(1):70-88. DOI: 10.1080/08952841.2012.638873. PubMed: 22256879

[25] Johnston O, Reilly J, Kremer J. Women's experiences of appearance concern and body control across the lifespan: Challenging accepted wisdom. Journal of Health Psychology. 2004;**9**(3):397-410. DOI: 10.1177/1359105304042349. PubMed: 15117539

[26] Mark Clarke LH. Older women's perceptions of ideal body weights: The tensions between health and appearance motivations for weight loss. Ageing and Society. 2002;**22**(06):751-773. DOI: 10.1017/S0144686X02008905

[27] Tunaley JR, Walsh S, Nicolson P. I'm not bad for my age: The meaning of body size and eating in the lives of older women. Ageing and Society. 1999;**19**(06):741-759

[28] Liechty T, Yarnal CM. The role of body image in older women's leisure. Journal of Leisure Research. 2010;**42**(3):443-467

[29] Bytheway B, Johnson J. The sight of age. The body in everyday life. 1998:243-257. Book Chapter

[30] Wasylkiw L, Emms AA, Meuse R, Poirier KF. Are all models created equal? A content analysis of women in advertisements of fitness versus fashion magazines. Body Image. 2009;**6**(2):137-140. DOI: 10.1016/j.bodyim.2009.01.005. PubMed: 19237328

[31] Banister EM. Women's midlife experience of their changing bodies. Qualitative Health Research. 1999;**9**(4):520-537. DOI: 10.1177/104973299129122045

[32] Twigg J, Majima S. Consumption and the constitution of age: Expenditure patterns on clothing, hair and cosmetics among post-war baby boomers. Journal of Aging Studies. 2014;**30**:23-32. DOI: 10.1016/j.jaging.2014.03.003. PubMed: 24984905

[33] Linder EC. Dance as a therapeutic intervention for the elderly. Educational Gerontology. 1982;**8**(2):167-174

[34] Cherniack P, Cherniack AR. The benefit of pets and animal-assisted therapy to the health of older individuals. Current Gerontology and Geriatrics Research. 2014;**2014**:623203. DOI: 10.1155/2014/623203. Epub 2014 Nov 16

[35] Sollami A, Gianferrari E, Alfieri M, Artioli G, Taffurelli C. Pet therapy: An effective strategy to care for the elderly? An experimental study in a nursing home. Acta Bio Medica. 2017;**88**(1-S): 25-31. DOI: 10.23750/abm.v88i1 -S.6281

[36] Hartung F-M, Renner B. Social curiosity and Gossip: Related but different drives of social Functioning. PLoS One;**8**(7):e69996. DOI: 10:1371/journale.pone.0069996

[37] Denecke K, Bamidis P, Bond C, Gabarron E, Househ M, Lau AY, Mayer MA, Merolli M, Hansen M.Ethical issues of social media usage in healthcare. Yearb Med Inform. Aug 13, 2015;**10**(1):137-147. DOI: 10.15265/IY-2015-001

[38] Arlati S, Colombo V, Spoladore D, Greci L, Pedroli E, et al. A social virtual reality-based application for the physical and cognitive training of the elderly at home sensors. 2019;**19**(2):261

[39] Savaskan E, Summermatter D, Schroeder C, Schächinger H. Memory deficits for facial identity in patients with amnestic mild cognitive impairment (MCI). PLoS One. 2018;**13**(4):e0195693. DOI: 10.1371/journal.pone.0195693. eCollection 2018

[40] The Black Dog. Department of Mental Health and substance abuse. World Health Organization 2015. Illustrator and author Matthew Johnstone; 2015

[41] Li CJ, Wang CH, Lin CF. An experience applying life review and resilience to a geriatric patient with functional limitations and depression. Hu li za zhi The journal of nursing. 2019;**66**(1):115-122. DOI: 10.6224/JN.201902_66(1).14

Section 2

Developments in Dementia

Chapter 3

Primary Prevention of Alzheimer's Disease (AD)

Ettore Bergamini and Gabriella Cavallini

Abstract

Alzheimer dementia (AD) is a complex, aging-associated disease whose effects on the brain (an organ made up by nonreplaceable cells) are devastating. Disease is not curable, but progress in pathobiology shows that intervention on aging can make primary prevention of AD feasible. According to the amyloid-cascade hypothesis, mechanisms of AD include: an age-related alteration of free radical metabolism in membranes, leading to a higher yield in the toxic Aβ1-42 peptide and an overwhelming impact on the weaker repair mechanisms of the aging cells. The proposed intervention on aging with anti-AD effects includes a daily assumption of antioxidants (red wine polyphenols enriched with resveratrol), a reinforcement of membrane antioxidant defenses by the assumption of polyunsaturated fatty acids at the first meal after fasting, and an enhancement of cell repair function (at the proteasome and autophagy level by an intermittent feeding regimen and physical exercise plus the assumption of antilipolytic agents during time of fasting). The beneficial effects of diet and physical activity on the endogenous production of protective nerve growth factors are magnified by an enriched environment. Treatment has already been started on healthy individuals at a higher risk of AD in the city of Volterra.

Keywords: Alzheimer's disease, proteasome, autophagy, antioxidants, PUFAs, APP, cholesterol, antilipolytic drugs, calorie restriction, physical exercise, brain plasticity, nerve growth factors

1. Introduction

Like many other degenerative diseases, AD is an irreversible and progressive cerebropathy, the cause of one of the most common types of dementia affecting the elderly. It is a brain disorder characterized by the accumulation of two main protein aggregates, senile plaques and neurofibrillary tangles, leading to a progressive neuronal degeneration. It causes death after years of disability, progressive loss of memory, inability to perform normal daily activities, and, finally, dementia. The senile plaques are generated by the deposition in human brain of fibrils of the β-amyloid peptide (Aβ), a fragment derived from the proteolytic processing of the amyloid precursor protein (APP). There is evidence that oxidative stress might be the main factor that turns APP into a proteolytically processable substrate. The neurofibrillary tangles (NFTs) are seen as a compact filamentous network formed by paired helical filaments (PHFs), whose major component is a hyperphosphorylated Tau protein. Two main protein kinases appear to be involved in the anomalous tau phosphorylation: the cyclin-dependent kinase Cdk5 and glycogen synthase kinase GSK3. Dysfunction of the ubiquitin-proteasome system may be the cause [1] possibly together with a secondary failure of the engulfed lysosomal degradation resulting in apoptosis. Pathology is a consequence of the extensive neuronal death, and when it manifests clinically, it is already incurable. Human, social, and health costs of this incurable disease are immense. It is highly desirable indeed an effective primary prevention to postpone the appearance of the debilitating manifestations, hopefully to the time of death.

2. Biological aging: Is it a major risk or the basic causative factor for neurodegeneration?

Age is the main factor in major debilitating and life-threatening conditions, including cancer, cardiovascular disease, diabetes, and neurodegeneration, all of which are therefore increasing in prevalence [2]. Nowadays almost all can make it to the old and nobody can say anymore that reaching old age is a fortune, and between those who should solve social and health problems of older people prevails the old slogan "old age is not a disease." For many scholars, however, modern scientific discoveries confirm the deductions of ancient philosophers: all living beings, without exception, would be affected by an innate chronic degenerative disease, we call it aging, characterized by having an incubation period as long as be compatible with the reproductive success of the species. If aging is a disease and not a simple disability and disease risk factor, it is not surprising that the diseases associated with it (cancer, neurodegeneration, atherosclerosis, diabetes, etc.) can be regarded as signs or easily preventable complications, all together, by fighting the underlying disease. The prescription is simple but hard to follow a sober physically active lifestyle; to eat fruits, vegetables, fish, and little red meat; to take food after having been hungry for a few hours; to take supplements rich in polyunsaturated fatty acids (PUFAs) after dinner regularly; and to make good use of all functions of all organs of our body, including brain. This is exactly what cardiologists, diabetologists, oncologists, and neurologists all recommend for primary prevention. Understanding exactly the causes of aging and of all age-associated diseases may help to tackle the growing problem of neurodegeneration. Free radicals are the root of all evil. They may be generated either by endogenous (metabolic) causes or by environmental factors, including pollution (living less than 50 m from a major traffic road may increase hazards ratio of incident dementia by a 10% [3] and even oral hygiene and chronic inflammation [4]). Perhaps, we should remind here the oxygen paradox: without oxygen we die in minutes; with oxygen we grow old and die [5]. Oxygen is actually slowly poisonous, and it just takes 75–100 years to kill us, difference depending on how much we use and how we deal with it and repair the endogenous oxidative damage to protein, lipids, and (most important) DNA responsible for intrinsic aging, as well as the additional free radical-mediated damage from the inflammatory responses and environmental factors (e.g., ionizing radiation) [6]. It was computed that the oxygen consumption of human brain may be higher than 3 mL (i.e., about 1020 oxygen molecules)/g/min. In humans, over 99% of these molecules do generate water safely, but 10^{18} per min will produce free radicals, approximately 10^6 free radicals per cell per min. It was estimated that the number of oxidative hits to DNA in the human cell per day is about 10,000 and that DNA-repair enzymes efficiently remove 99.9% of the lesions formed so that only one oxidative lesion accumulate in the DNA of any cell every day. This is not nothing: it makes over 30,000 lesions in a long life [7]. Since there are about 20,000 genes in human cells, by the age of 100 years, all neurons may carry about two mutations a gene on the average. Why be surprised if over time cell functions are reduced?

3. Pathology of AD

With AD patients, the brain is smaller than normal and of reduced weight. A reduction of the thickness of the convolutions is evident. Atrophy is more evident in the temporal lobe, particularly in the parahippocampus, but also in the frontal and parietal regions. The occipital lobe and the motor cortex may be spared. Histologically, several major changes are recognized in AD. Amyloid, consisting of accumulations of Aβ peptide, is deposed in the cerebral cortex in the form of spherical deposits called senile plaques. Intraneuronal inclusions are formed in the cortical neurons, constituted by abnormal, often flame-shaped, bundles of filaments called neurofibrillary tangles, which occupy a large part of the neuronal cytoplasm, and are made up of a protein that binds to the microtubules, called tau protein. The processes of the cortical nerve cells diverge, twist, and dilate due to the accumulation of filaments in the form of tangles [8]. Changes are due to oxidative stress damage and to the relative failure of repair mechanisms at the molecular and subcellular (autophagy) level and result in the disruption of the neural network (**Table 1**). It is customary to distinguish two forms of AD. There is indeed a precocious rare form that occurs between 30 and 60 years, with a peak in the fifties, with a formation of the amyloidogenic peptide Aβ (1-42) from APP genetically favored by particular isoforms of presenilin 1 and 2 or of APP. The other form, sporadic, more frequent, late-onset (observed after age 65 with a frequency that increases with age) is due to the progressive increase in oxidative stress and decline with increasing age in mitochondrial and peroxisomal maintenance and in the efficiency of the mechanisms that neutralize free radicals and repair damage. This latter form might be postponed successfully to time of death by anti-aging interventions (nutrition, physical activity, damage repair, nerve growth factors).

4. The primary cause of AD and the roles of cholesterol and unsaturated fatty acids

It is obvious that native APP cannot be the ultimate substrate for γ-secretase trimming. Hence, both with the earlier and the later form of AD, the rate of Aβ

Mechanism of repair	Effects of the age-related decline
Molecular level	
DNA repair Proteasome Phospholipid repair	Accumulation of DNA lesion Accumulation of altered proteins Changes in polyunsaturated fatty acids
Subcellular Level	
Autophagy and lysosomal function	Accumulation of altered mitochondria Accumulation of protein aggregates Changes in membrane proteins and lipids
Cellular and tissue level	
Apoptosis	Accumulation of damaged, misfunctional cells in all tissues

There is evidence that the above-mentioned repair mechanisms are responsible for cleaning cells from any produced waste and for getting tissues rid of irreversibly altered cells. In younger persons, functions are redundant but progressively decline with increasing age, and may gradually fail in older persons resulting in the accumulation of "waste" in cells and tissues. On a healthy life, "waste" is the limiting factor for cell and tissue "cleaning" activities, but waste recognition-acuity co-varies with cell and body request for nutrients and repair. Function of all repair mechanisms are inducible (or suppressible) depending on life style. Benefits from healthy life style, diet restriction, and physical activity depend at least in part from the induction of repair mechanisms.

Table 1.
Effects of failure of repair mechanisms at the molecular, subcellular, and cellular level.

production from APP should depend on a higher production of the ultimate substrate, possibly by a posttranslational modification of the APP molecules, likely to be secondary to oxidative stress. Age-related changes in the machinery that protects membrane proteins from free radical-mediated injury might help to account for age dependency [9]. With regard to the higher production of Aβ (1-42) in AD patients, a displacement of the free radical-mediated attack from the wanted site in the APP molecule might account for the higher involvement of the β and γ secretase pathways and the higher yield in Aβ 1-42. The effect may be favored either by genetic factors and/or aging.

4.1 Role of cholesterol

Elevated cholesterol levels may be associated with a higher risk of AD [10]. Evidence was found suggesting an intimate connection between APP processing and lipid rafts [11]. An age-related increase in cholesterol and oxidized cholesterol products (namely 24-hydroxycholesterol and 27-hydroxycholesterol) was shown indeed to be increasingly associated with AD progression (brain levels are higher in AD patients, and levels of 24-hydroxycholesterol, 27-hydroxycholesterol and cholesterol in the cerebrospinal fluid appear to be useful biomarkers for the evaluation of mild cognitive impairment (MCI) and AD, together with Aβ42, total tau, and phospho-tau) [12]. It has been shown recently that higher total cholesterol levels in the blood are observed long before the clinical manifestation of MCI and AD in patients without psychiatric or somatic comorbidities and are independent of APOE genotype [13]. However, evidence was produced that changes in cholesterol metabolism in AD may not be the primary cause of the disease (see below): they may simply be a tightly associated sign with Aβ production by sharing a common cause (a higher intramembrane oxidative stress) (see below).

4.2 Role of polyunsaturated fatty acids (PUFAs)

PUFAs and their oxylipins may affect the onset of AD [14]. The administration of omega-3 fatty acids may cause a dose-dependent reduction of triglyceridemia and cholesterolemia and exert an antiatherogenic effect [15]. With regard to mechanisms, in view of the proposed protective role of unsaturated fatty acids in phospholipids against the free radical-mediated injury of membrane proteins [9], it should be mentioned that the distribution of unsaturation (the trap for unpaired electrons) across the membrane leaflets is not uniform, and minima (the least protected areas from oxidative stress) were observed close to the C-6 site (i.e., very close to the membrane exterior, to the phosphorylable site of HMGCoAR, and to the vulnerable site of APP) and at the C-15 and C-17 levels (closer to the free radical conductor dolichol) [16]. Quite interestingly, signal might help focus free radical-mediated injury on the right target; more interestingly, in ad-libitum-fed (shorter-lived) rats, is its recognizability that may fade on aging: the abundancy of double bonds near the C-6 site (but not at the C-15 and C-17) indeed appears to increase up to a doubling by age 24 months. Furthermore, this age-related change is prevented in part by nutritional anti-aging intervention [17]. Perhaps age-related changes in the production of Aβ1-42, in the activity of HMGCoA reductase, and in the PUFA content of membrane phospholipids are all somehow bound together and involved all in the risk of AD. As an additional comment, beneficial intervention on Aβ1-42 production may require the administration of antioxidants (e.g., polyphenols and resveratrol) to curb oxidative stress and of omega-3 fatty acids at a high dosage at the first good meal after fast (on the anabolic phase of metabolism) to counteract age-related changes in phospholipid unsaturated fatty acids and increase membrane resistance to oxidative stress. An enhancement of the membrane turnover rate may be useful (e.g., by dietary restriction and/or pharmacological stimulation of autophagy) [18].

5. The pathogenesis of AD

The hypothesis of the amyloid cascade attributes to beta-amyloid, the responsibility of all cases of AD, and considers the tau pathology and other degenerative changes secondary to the Aβ pathology. Indeed, the extracellular accumulation of Aβ, a hallmark of AD, produces ROS, including hydrogen peroxide (H_2O_2) in the presence of Fe^{3+}or Cu^{2+} [19, 20]. The amyloid β-peptide responsible for AD is generated within the transmembrane domain (TMD) of a C-terminal fragment of the amyloid β protein-precursor (APP CTFβ) by the proteolytic action of the γ-secretase complex [21]. Very interestingly, it was shown that some mutation(s) that promote destabilization of TMD helix might affect the length of the accumulated Aβ species and the ratio of the toxic Aβ42 to the safer Aβ40 peptide and may result in a young-onset AD [22]. Hence, the speculation may be invited that a free radical-induced modification in (some) amino acids of APP close to the C-6 carbon of phospholipid fatty acids might have a similar effect and enhance amyloid deposition. With regard to disease progression, many different active factors in sequence would determine timing of neuronal damage and symptom development, such as: (1) an overproduction of the toxic Aβ peptide (1-42) for genetic reasons and/or decrease in the quality of the antioxidant device of the membranes, (2) an ensuing increase in Aβ excretion in the oligomeric form may concentrate the redox-active copper at neuronal membranes before stacking in amyloid fibrils to form an ROS generating complex, (3) oxidative stress may be enhanced with an ensuing increase in lipid peroxidation and di-tyrosine formation, and (4) inflammation and activation of the microglia, which may further increase free radical generation, spread lytic enzymes, and cause cytotoxicity and anticipation of apoptotic neuronal death [23].

6. AD-associated changes in cholesterol metabolism

Abnormal cholesterol metabolism is an established feature of AD: levels of cholesterol are increased in MCI subjects and levels of 24-hydroxycholesterol and 27-hydroxycholesterol are elevated compared to controls both in AD and MCI subjects [24]. It appears that the rate of cholesterol production may be boosted by a free radical attack via a constitutive activation of HMGCoA-reductase, the rate-limiting step in sterol biosynthesis. Mechanism was clarified by Bergamini group in Pisa in cooperation with Trentalance group in Rome: in the rat, a free radical attack may prevent AMP-dependent protein kinase from phosphorylating a serine residue close to the C-terminus of HMGCoA reductase, Ser 872 with human enzyme [25, 26]. It has been proposed by several authors that higher cholesterol may disturb the lipid raft domains in various membrane organelles and affect the functioning of α, β, and γ secretases as well as APP itself and the production of Aβ 42; and that by converse, the toxicity of Aβ may be produced, in part, by disturbing the composition of the lipid raft domains in which they reside [27, 28]. Both with in vitro experiments and with animal models, statins strongly lowered blood cholesterol and reduced the levels of Aβ peptides, Aβ 42 and A β40 [29, 30]. However, a statistically significant correlation between two events does not necessarily imply the existence of a causal link: an alternative explanation is that the events share a common cause. This might be the case here: aging is known to lower antioxidant defenses, and any increase in oxidative stress either in vitro (e.g., by UV radiation of isolated rat liver cells) or in vivo (by chronic deprivation either of vitamin E or PUFA) may cause the constitutive increase in HMGCoA reductase and deregulate cholesterol synthesis [26, 31].

7. Alzheimer's disease: treatment or prevention strategies?

The pharmacological treatments for AD can be divided into two categories: symptomatic treatments such as acetylcholinesterase inhibitors and N-methyl-D-aspartate (NMDA) receptor antagonists and etiology-based treatments such as secretase inhibitors, amyloid binders, and tau therapies [32].

Despite significant investments in therapeutic drug discovery programs, no drugs to alter the course of disease have been found so far. Only four drugs with cholinergic (donepezil, galantamine, rivastigmine) or glutamatergic activity (Memantine) are currently approved and marketed for the treatment of AD-associated dementia, and their utility is very limited; several trials on inhibitors of γ-secretase and β-secretase have been discontinued; the available drug treatments of AD are merely symptomatic and unsatisfactory, and only minor benefits are obtained even if therapy is started at a very early time [33]. By the way, the physiological function of the amyloidogenic peptide has not been clarified yet, though it may be synchronized with life history [34].

In conclusion, no effective therapy is available to cure AD so far, and attention had to be shifted to the primary prevention of the disease. It was realized indeed that there is an extremely long, symptom-free prodromal phase in the path toward dementia in which deficits in synaptic density and plasticity are the principal alteration [35]. As an additional comment, better diagnostic tools and earlier diagnosis are needed (earlier timing is an important factor for the success rate of intervention), and novel strategies toward primary intervention may be wanted [36].

Problems in primary prevention were tackled recently. Qiu et al. [37] stressed the potential risk roles of vascular risk factors and disorders (e.g., cigarette smoking, midlife high blood pressure and obesity, diabetes, and cerebrovascular lesions) and the possible beneficial roles of psychosocial factors (e.g., high education, active social engagement, physical exercise, and mentally stimulating activity) in the pathogenetic process and clinical manifestation of the dementing disorders. Paillard-Borg et al. [38] showed that the participation in activities (mental, physical, or social activity) can retard the onset of dementia significantly (a 17 months' delay was seen in mean age at dementia onset between an inactive group and the most active group).

It may be worthwhile to remind here that the primary risk factor for AD is old age and that the prevalence of AD and other age-related dementias increases with increasing age [2]. It is very surprising, indeed, that little attention has been given so far to benefits from the most effective antiaging interventions (dietary restriction and physical activity) on the age of onset of neurodegeneration [39].

Antiaging diet restriction is known to be the most effective intervention that retards aging and extends lifespan and health span. Effects are known to involve the activation of macroautophagy, a cell repair mechanism [40] that can be intensified by the administration of antilipolytic agents during fasting to safely improve cell housekeeping and boost the benefits of caloric restriction [41]. Physical exercise, which is available at low cost and largely free of adverse effects, is another powerful antiaging strategy that can influence, at least partly, most of the hallmarks of biological aging [42]. It is known that greater levels of physical activity are associated with decreased risk of a future diagnosis of MCI or AD [43], extend longevity, and reduce the risk of physical disability and may be an important adjunct to pharmacological treatment of AD [44].

Looking at mechanisms, it appears that dietary restriction and physical exercise share common neuroprotective mechanisms and should be included both in primary prevention of AD to increase the quality of nerve cells and oppose neurodegeneration and apoptosis (the third item in the **Table 1**, a repair mechanism harmful to brain) and give synergic support in a "train body and brain" program aimed to enhance neurotrophic antiapoptotic signals and defer or suppress neuron misfunctioning and death [45].

Antiaging diet restriction improves metabolism and promotes rejuvenation (by stimulating autophagy) of visceral organs that talk to brain via the vagus nerve and spinal afferent nerves [46]. Physical exercise improves metabolism and promotes rejuvenation of the lean body mass by the process of autophagy, which is very active in skeletal muscle and more intense when strenuous exercise is performed in the fasted state [47] and helps communication of the exercising muscle with the brain via increase in the discharge frequency of thinly myelinated (Group III) and unmyelinated (Group IV) nerve fibers [48]. Under these conditions, physical exercise is good both for physical health and mental health and abilities, and constitutes a practical neuroprotective strategy that provides a remarkable protection against brain insults of different etiology and anatomy [49].

Quite interesting, it has been clarified that dietary restriction and physical exercise share also common neuroprotective metabolic mechanism: the increased availability to brain of 3-hydroxybutyrate and an ensuing endogenous production of the brain-derived-neurotrophic-factor BDNF [50], and thus, both shelter the aging brain from memory loss and neurodegeneration, ameliorate mitochondrial function, and reduce the expression of apoptotic and inflammatory mediators [51]. As an additional evidence: both treatments safely modulate the endogenous production of BDNF, a neurotrophin that is vital to the survival, growth, and maintenance of neurons in key brain circuits involved in emotional and cognitive function [52, 53]. As an additional benefit, sustained levels of physical exercise together with dietary intervention may increase brain uptake of physiologically relevant neuroprotective trophic factors, such as IGF-I [49].

In conclusion, both (dietary and physical) interventions should be included in primary prevention of AD to increase quality of nerve cells and oppose neurodegeneration and apoptosis to implement reported programs aimed to enhance neurotrophic antiapoptotic signals and defer or suppress neuron misfunctioning and death.

8. The "train body and brain" protocol for a primary intervention on AD in the city of Volterra (Tuscany, Italy)

In view of the continuing increase in the prevalence of dementia to a magnitude growing to emergency [54, 55], a free of charge program to train people at higher risk of disease has been started in the Italian city of Volterra. Since AD is an aging-associated multifaceted disease that is hard to treat by single-modal treatment, a corresponding multifaceted preventive approach was included in a teaching program on how to counteract in practice the effects of biological and pathological aging on human body and brain.

Program includes activation of the global antioxidant defense system in order to attenuate the AD-causative oxidative stress, improvement of the function of the free radical conducting mechanism responsible for membrane resistance to oxidative stress, reinforcement of cell repair mechanisms at the molecular and subcellular level by dietary and physical intervention, and targeted high-intensity training of cognitive brain functions to boost the induction of neurotrophic factors by the physiological mechanism. Here, a few details on protocol are given.

a. Strengthening antioxidant defenses by nutritional intervention. It is said that the efficiency of antioxidant defenses may be boosted by eating the colors in the peel of fruits and vegetables that are known to contain complex mixtures of polyphenols and other phytochemicals. (e.g., polyphenols in blueberries and red grapes and wine [56]; epigallocatechin-3-gallate in green tea [57]; total phenolic, flavonoids, and flavonols in pomegranate [58, 59]). Red wine is particularly rich in specific polyphenolic compounds that appear to affect the biological processes of AD and Parkinson's disease, such as quercetin, myricetin, catechins, tannins, anthocyanidins, resveratrol, and ferulic acid. Indeed, there is now a consistent body of in vitro and in vivo data on the neuroprotective activity of red wine polyphenols [60], and it is known that effects may be boosted by adding more resveratrol [61]. Obviously, to enjoy optimum benefits, participants are taught to assume phytochemicals in a way to ensure protection throughout the day.

b. Increasing the resistance of cell membranes to oxidative stress. In order to get a better resistance to ROS-induced damage to brain and prevent from neurodegeneration and neuronal apoptosis, participants are instructed to a timed assumption of omega-3-rich fish oil. PUFAs are essential to control oxidative damage to neurons [62] when they are incorporated in the phospholipid molecules as a part in the proposed antioxidant machinery that protects membrane proteins from peroxidation (**Figure 1**) (On the contrary, free PUFAs are very sensitive to a free radical attack and ready to peroxidation.) To get full benefit from supplement, participants are requested to take pills at the first good meal after the long time of fasting, when chances to be incorporated in membrane phospholipids are paramount [63].

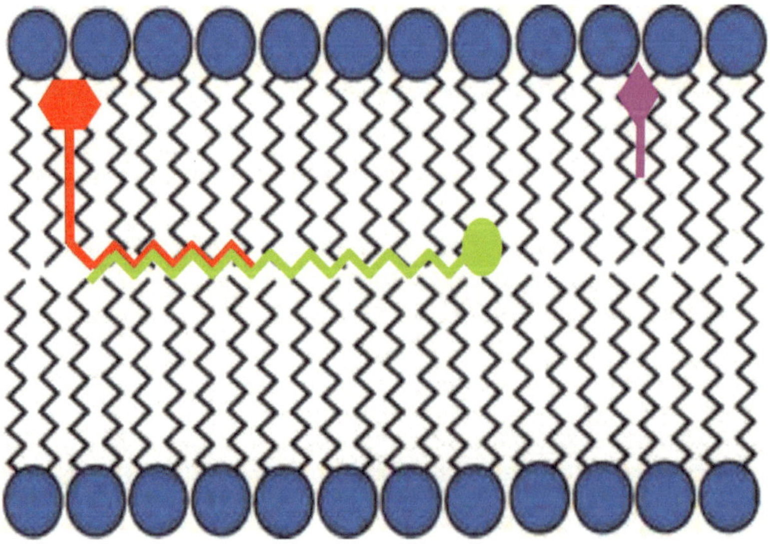

Figure 1.
Model of the membrane antioxidant machinery based on the proposed locations of dolichol (disc, green), ubiquinone (hexagon, red), and vitamin E (rhomb, pink) (see Cathcart et al. [69]; Sharma et al. [70]).

c. Promoting cell cleaning and rejuvenation. It is done by teaching participants in practice how to eat a healthy calorie-restricted diet and to make aerobic physical exercise during fasting. It is known indeed that calorie restriction is the most robust antiaging intervention known so far [64], and that benefit comes from the alternation of a long time of fasting and good meal (twice a week, participants spend a great part of their time in a state of fasting) [65] in order to get cells free of altered ROS-hypergenerating organelles in older cells [66, 67]. Good maintenance will be finalized later, thanks to a good meal. If needed, benefit might be magnified by taking a pill of an antilipolytic drug on the time of fasting [41]. Benefits of protocol might be monitored noninvasively by the assay of the urinary excretion of 8-hydroxy-2′-deoxyguanosine, a recently recommended biomarker for monitoring oxidative status over time [68].

d. A targeted high-intensity training of cognitive brain functions. In addition to the previously described interventions on diet and physical activity, the mental and the social activity protocols tested by Paillard-Borg et al. [38] are being practiced. In view of the results obtained by Dahlgren et al. [51], high intensity interval training (HIIT) and memory training using the PEAK brain training app are included in the protocol.

9. Conclusion

A dynamic antiaging nutritional and physical intervention protocol including enriched living conditions is described useful to prevent the appearance of aging-associated AD. Treatment is already granted for free to the citizens of the city of Volterra known to be at higher risk of AD (relatives of AD patients and persons with mild cognitive impairment, likely to progress to clinically probable AD at a considerably accelerated rate compared with healthy age-matched individuals) to teach them how to counteract and retard the disease. Treatment was designed to delay biological aging and empower adult brain plasticity in order to retard the progress of brain aging and associated diseases. It includes a daily assumption of antioxidants (red wine polyphenols enriched with resveratrol), a reinforcement of membrane antioxidant defenses by the timed assumption of polyunsaturated fatty acids, and an enhancement of cell repair function at the molecular and subcellular level by an intermittent feeding regimen and physical exercise, whose efficiency is empowered by the pharmacological intensification of autophagy by an antilipolytic drug (Acipimox) taken at a very low dosage while fasting. The beneficial effects on neurodegeneration are magnified by living an enriched environment. The effectiveness of the treatment will be detected by comparison with the expected frequencies of disease appearance.

Acknowledgements

Research is a part in the "train body and brain" project organized and supported by Volterra Research Foundation, Rotary District 2071, and Alberto Sordi Association, Rome, under the patronage of the city of Volterra. The project was born to give school-age citizens the most modern information on how to achieve an effective primary prevention of all chronic age-associated diseases, including neurodegenerative diseases, and to offer adult people at higher risk of Alzheimer's disease (relatives of patients and patients with MCI) a free service of practical education on how to prevent and slow down the progression of the disease. The first goal is achieved by donating to high school students a pdf entitled "How to keep in shape, preventing diseases and defending good health" (available on the site www.fondazionevolterraricerche.org). The "train body and brain" project was approved by the Istituto Superiore di Sanità and has patronage of the Italian Ministry of Education.

Conflict of interest

The authors disclose no conflicts.

Author details

Ettore Bergamini[1,2*] and Gabriella Cavallini[3]

1 University Campus Biomedico, Roma, Italy

2 Volterra Ricerche Onlus Foundation, Volterra, Italy

3 Interdepartmental Research Centre on Biology and Pathology of Aging, University of Pisa, Italy

*Address all correspondence to: ettore.bergamini@gmail.com

References

[1] Tai HC, Serrano-Pozo A, Hashimoto T, Frosch MP, Spires-Jones TL, Hyman BT. The synaptic accumulation of hyperphosphorylated tau oligomers in Alzheimer disease is associated with dysfunction of the ubiquitin-proteasome system. The American Journal of Pathology. 2012;**181**:1426-1435. DOI: 10.1016/j.ajpath.2012.06.033

[2] Niccoli T, Partridge L. Ageing as a risk factor for disease. Current Biology. 2012;**22**:R741-R752. DOI: 10.1016/j.cub.2012.07.024

[3] Chen H, Kwong JC, Copes R, Tu K, Villeneuve PJ, van Donkelaar A, et al. Living near major roads and the incidence of dementia, Parkinson's disease, and multiple sclerosis: A population-based cohort study. Lancet. 2017;**389**:718-726. DOI: 10.1016/S0140-6736(16)32399-6

[4] Singhrao SK, Harding A, Poole S, Kesavalu L, Crean S. Porphyromonas gingivalis periodontal infection and its putative links with Alzheimer's disease. Mediators of Inflammation. 2015;**2015**:137357. DOI: 10.1155/2015/137357

[5] Davies KJ. The oxygen paradox, oxidative stress, and ageing. Archives of Biochemistry and Biophysics. 2016;**595**:28-32. DOI: 10.1016/j.abb.2015.11.015

[6] Davies JMS, Cillard J, Friguet B, Cadenas E, Cadet J, Cayce R, et al. The oxygen paradox, the French paradox, and age-related diseases. Geroscience. 2017;**39**:499-550. DOI: 10.1007/s11357-017-0002-y

[7] Ames BN, Shigenaga MK. Oxidants are a major contributor to aging. Annals of the New York Academy of Sciences. 1992;**663**:85-96. DOI: 10.1111/j.1749-6632.1992.tb38652.x

[8] Stevens A, Lowe J, Scott I. Core Pathology. 3rd ed. Edinburgh: Mosby Elsevier; 2009

[9] Bergamini E, Bizzarri R, Cavallini G, Cerbai B, Chiellini E, Donati A, et al. Ageing and oxidative stress: A role for dolichol in the antioxidant machinery of cell membranes? Journal of Alzheimer's Disease. 2004;**6**:129-135. DOI: 10.3233/JAD-2004-6204

[10] Xue-Shan Z, Juan P, Qi W, Zhong R, Li-Hong P, Zhi-Han T, et al. Imbalanced cholesterol metabolism in Alzheimer's disease. Clinica Chimica Acta. 2016;**456**:107-114. DOI: 10.1016/j.cca.2016.02.024

[11] Cheng H, Vetrivel KS, Gong P, Meckler X, Parent A, Thinakaran G. Mechanisms of disease: New therapeutic strategies for Alzheimer's disease-targeting APP processing in lipid rafts. Nature Clinical Practice. Neurology. 2007;**3**:374-382

[12] Wang HL, Wang YY, Liu XG, Kuo SH, Liu N, Song QY, et al. Cholesterol, 24-hydroxycholesterol, and 27-hydroxycholesterol as surrogate biomarkers in cerebrospinal fluid in mild cognitive impairment and Alzheimer's disease: A meta-analysis. Journal of Alzheimer's Disease. 2016;**51**:45-55. DOI: 10.3233/JAD-150734

[13] Toro P, Degen C, Pierer M, Gustafson D, Schröder J, Schönknecht P. Cholesterol in mild cognitive impairment and Alzheimer's disease in a birth cohort over 14 years. European Archives of Psychiatry and Clinical Neuroscience. 2014;**264**:485-492. DOI: 10.1007/s00406-013-0468-2

[14] Devassy JG, Leng S, Gabbs M, Monirujjaman M, Aukema HM. Omega-3 polyunsaturated fatty acids and oxylipins in neuroinflammation and management of Alzheimer disease.

Advances in Nutrition. 2016;7:905-916. DOI: 10.3945/an.116.012187

[15] Gladine C, Newman JW, Durand T, Pedersen TL, Galano JM, Demougeot C, et al. Lipid profiling following intake of the omega 3 fatty acid DHA identifies the peroxidized metabolites F4-neuroprostanes as the best predictors of atherosclerosis prevention. PLoS One. 2014;**9**:e89393. DOI: 10.1371/journal.pone.0089393

[16] Tamburini I, Quartacci MF, Izzo R, Bergamini E. Effects of dietary restriction on age-related changes in the phospholipid fatty acid composition of various rat tissues. Aging Clinical and Experimental Research. 2004;**16**: 425-431. DOI: 10.1007/BF03327396

[17] Tamburini I. Invecchiamento e stress ossidativo: Effetti dell'invecchiamento, di trattamenti anti-invecchiamento e di modulazioni acute e croniche dello stress ossidativo su molecule perossidabili lipofile di membrane [PhD thesis]. Pisa: University of Pisa; 2006

[18] Bergamini E. Targets for antiageing drugs. Expert Opinion on Therapeutic Targets. 2005;**9**:77-82

[19] Huang X, Cuajungco MP, Atwood CS, Hartshorn MA, Tyndall JD, Hanson GR, et al. Cu(II) potentiation of alzheimer abeta neurotoxicity. Correlation with cell-free hydrogen peroxide production and metal reduction. The Journal of Biological Chemistry. 1999;**274**:37111-37116. DOI: 10.1074/jbc.274.52.37111

[20] Nadal RC, Rigby SE, Viles JH. Amyloid beta-Cu^{2+} complexes in both monomeric and fibrillar forms do not generate H_2O_2 catalytically but quench hydroxyl radicals. Biochemistry. 2008;**47**:11653-11664. DOI: 10.1021/bi8011093

[21] Fernandez MA, Biette KM, Dolios G, Seth D, Wang R, Wolfe MS. Transmembrane substrate determinants for γ-secretase processing of APP CTFβ. Biochemistry. 2016;**55**:5675-5688. DOI: 10.1021/acs.biochem.6b00718

[22] Liu CY, Ohki Y, Tomita T, Osawa S, Reed BR, Jagust W, et al. Two novel mutations in the first transmembrane domain of presenilin1 cause young-onset Alzheimer's disease. Journal of Alzheimer's Disease. 2017;**58**:1035-1041. DOI: 10.3233/JAD-161203

[23] Bergamini E. Autophagy: A cell repair mechanism that retards ageing and age-associated diseases and can be intensified pharmacologically. Molecular Aspects of Medicine. 2006;**27**:403-410. DOI: 10.1016/j.mam.2006.08.001

[24] Chang T-Y, Yamauchi Y, Hasan MT, Chang C. Cellular cholesterol homeostasis and Alzheimer's disease. Journal of Lipid Research. 2017;**58**: 2239-2254. DOI: 10.1194/jlr.R075630

[25] Clarke PR, Hardie DG. Regulation of HMG-CoA reductase: Identification of the site phosphorylated by the AMP-activated protein kinase in vitro and in intact rat liver. The EMBO Journal. 1990;**9**:2439-2446

[26] Pallottini V, Martini C, Pascolini A, Cavallini G, Gori Z, Bergamini E, et al. 3-Hydroxy-3-methylglutaryl coenzyme A reductase deregulation and age-related hypercholesterolemia: A new role for ROS. Mechanisms of Ageing and Development. 2005;**126**:845-851. DOI: 10.1016/j.mad.2005.02.009

[27] Vetrivel KS, Thinakaran G. Membrane rafts in Alzheimer's disease beta-amyloid production. Biochimica et Biophysica Acta. 2010;**1801**:860-867. DOI: 10.1016/j.bbalip.2010.03.007

[28] Barrett PJ, Song Y, Van Horn WD, Hustedt EJ, Schafer JM, Hadziselimovic A, et al. The amyloid precursor protein has a flexible transmembrane domain and binds cholesterol. Science. 2012;**336**:1168-1171. DOI: 10.1126/science.1219988

[29] Fassbender K, Simons M, Bergmann C, Stroick M, Lutjohann D, Keller P, et al. Simvastatin strongly reduces levels of Alzheimer's disease beta-amyloid peptides Abeta 42 and Abeta 40 in vitro and in vivo. Proceedings of the National Academy of Sciences of the United States of America. 2001;**98**:5856-5861. DOI: 10.1073/pnas.081620098

[30] Shinohara M, Sato N, Kurinami H, Takeuchi D, Takeda S, Shimamura M, et al. Reduction of brain beta-amyloid (Abeta) by fluvastatin, a hydroxymethylglutaryl-CoA reductase inhibitor, through increase in degradation of amyloid precursor protein C-terminal fragments (APP-CTFs) and Abeta clearance. The Journal of Biological Chemistry. 2010;**285**:22091-22102. DOI: 10.1074/jbc.M110.102277

[31] Pallottini V, Martini C, Cavallini G, Bergamini E, Mustard KJ, Hardie DG, et al. Age-related HMG-CoA reductase deregulation depends on ROS-induced p38 activation. Mechanisms of Ageing and Development. 2007;**128**:688-695. DOI: 10.1016/j.mad.2007.10.001

[32] Mendiola-Precoma J, Berumen LC, Padilla K, Garcia-Alcocer G. Therapies for prevention and treatment of Alzheimer's disease. BioMed Research International. 2016;**2016**:2589276. DOI: 10.1155/2016/2589276

[33] Graham WV, Bonito-Oliva A, Sakmar TP. Update on Alzheimer's disease therapy and prevention strategies. Annual Review of Medicine. 2017;**68**:413-430. DOI: 10.1146/annurev-med-042915-103753

[34] Maldonado TA, Jones RE, Norris DO. Distribution of beta-amyloid and amyloid precursor protein in the brain of spawning (senescent) salmon: A natural, brain-aging model. Brain Research. 2000;**858**:237-251. DOI: 10.1016/S0006-8993(99)02328-8

[35] Dubois B, Hampel H, Feldman HH, Scheltens P, Aisen P, Andrieu S, et al. Proceedings of the meeting of the international working group (IWG) and the American Alzheimer's Association on "the preclinical state of AD"; July 23, 2015; Washington DC, USA. Preclinical Alzheimer's disease: Definition, natural history, and diagnostic criteria. Alzheimer's & Dementia. 2016;**12**:292-323. DOI: 10.1016/j.jalz.2016.02.002

[36] Tan CC, Yu JT, Tan L. Biomarkers for preclinical Alzheimer's disease. Journal of Alzheimer's Disease. 2014;**42**:1051-1069. DOI: 10.3233/JAD-140843

[37] Qiu C, Kivipelto M, von Strauss E. Epidemiology of Alzheimer's disease: Occurrence, determinants, and strategies toward intervention. Dialogues in Clinical Neuroscience. 2009;**11**:111-128

[38] Paillard-Borg S, Fratiglioni L, Xu W, Winblad B, Wang HX. An active lifestyle postpones dementia onset by more than one year in very old adults. Journal of Alzheimer's Disease. 2012;**31**:835-842. DOI: 10.3233/JAD-2012-120724

[39] Blagosklonny MV. Prospective treatment of age-related diseases by slowing down aging. The American Journal of Pathology. 2012;**181**:1142-1146. DOI: 10.1016/j.ajpath.2012.06.024

[40] Bergamini E, Cavallini G, Donati A, Gori Z. The role of macroautophagy in the ageing process, anti-ageing intervention and age-associated diseases. The International Journal

of Biochemistry & Cell Biology. 2004;**36**:2392-2404. DOI: 10.1016/j.biocel.2004.05.007

[41] Bergamini E. Searching for the fountain of autophagy-dependent youth: Ettore Bergamini. Interview by Daniel J. Klionsky. Autophagy. 2012;**8**: 1169-1174. DOI: 10.4161/auto.20788

[42] Fiuza-Luces C, Garatachea N, Berger NA, Lucia A. Exercise is the real polypill. Physiology (Bethesda). 2013;**28**:330-358. DOI: 10.1152/physiol.00019.2013

[43] Schlosser Covell GE, Hoffman-Snyder CR, Wellik KE, Woodruff BK, Geda YE, Caselli RJ, et al. Physical activity level and future risk of mild cognitive impairment or dementia: A critically appraised topic. The Neurologist. 2015;**19**:89-91. DOI: 10.1097/NRL.0000000000000013

[44] Aguirre LE, Villareal DT. Physical exercise as therapy for frailty. Nestlé Nutrition Institute Workshop Series. 2015;**83**:83-92. DOI: 10.1159/000382065

[45] Sale A, Berardi N, Maffei L. Environment and brain plasticity: Towards an endogenous pharmacotherapy. Physiological Reviews. 2014;**94**:189-234. DOI: 10.1152/physrev.00036.2012

[46] Spencer NJ, Zagorodnyuk V, Brookes SJ, Hibberd T. Spinal afferent nerve endings in visceral organs: Recent advances. American Journal of Physiology Gastrointestinal and Liver Physiology. 2016;**311**:G1056-G1063. DOI: 10.1152/ajpgi.00319.2016

[47] Martin-Rincon M, Morales-Alamo D, Calbet JAL. Exercise-mediated modulation of autophagy in skeletal muscle. Scandinavian Journal of Medicine & Science in Sports. 2018;**28**:772-781. DOI: 10.1111/sms.12945

[48] Amann M. Significance of group III and IV muscle afferents for the endurance exercising human. Clinical and Experimental Pharmacology & Physiology. 2012;**39**:831-835. DOI: 10.1111/j.1440-1681.2012.05681.x

[49] Carro E, Trejo JL, Busiguina S, Torres-Aleman I. Circulating insulin-like growth factor I mediates the protective effects of physical exercise against brain insults of different etiology and anatomy. The Journal of Neuroscience. 2001;**21**:5678-5684. DOI: 10.1523/JNEUROSCI.21-15-05678.2001

[50] Marosi K, Kim SW, Moehl K, Scheibye-Knudsen M, Cheng A, Cutler R, et al. 3-Hydroxybutyrate regulates energy metabolism and induces BDNF expression in cerebral cortical neurons. Journal of Neurochemistry. 2016;**139**:769-781. DOI: 10.1111/jnc.13868

[51] Dahlgren K, Gibas KJ. Ketogenic diet, high intensity interval training (HIIT) and memory training in the treatment of mild cognitive impairment: A case study. Diabetes and Metabolic Syndrome: Clinical Research and Reviews. 2018;**12**:819-822. DOI: 10.1016/j.dsx.2018.04.031

[52] Cherif A, Roelands B, Meeusen R, Chamari K. Effects of intermittent fasting, caloric restriction, and Ramadan intermittent fasting on cognitive performance at rest and during exercise in adults. Sports Medicine. 2016;**46**:35-47. DOI: 10.1007/s40279-015-0408-6

[53] Huang T, Larsen KT, Ried-Larsen M, Møller NC, Andersen LB. The effects ofphysical activity and exercise on brain-derived neurotrophic factor in healthy humans: A review. Scandinavian Journal of Medicine & Science in Sports. 2014;**24**:1-10. DOI: 10.1111/sms.12069

[54] von Strauss E, Viitanen M, De Ronchi D, Winblad B, Fratiglioni L. Aging and the occurrence of dementia: Findings from a

population-based cohort with a large sample of nonagenarians. Archives of Neurology. 1999;**56**:587-592. DOI: 10.1001/archneur.56.5.587

[55] Corrada MM, Brookmeyer R, Berlau D, Paganini-Hill A, Kawas CH. Prevalence of dementia after age 90: Results from the 90+ study. Neurology. 2008;**71**:337-343. DOI: 10.1212/01.wnl.0000310773.65918.cd

[56] Li YR, Li S, Lin CC. Effect of resveratrol and pterostilbene on ageing and longevity. BioFactors. 2018;**44**: 69-82. DOI: 10.1002/biof.1400

[57] Cascella M, Bimonte S, Muzio MR, Schiavone V, Cuomo A. The efficacy of Epigallocatechin-3-gallate (green tea) in the treatment of Alzheimer's disease: An overview of pre-clinical studies and translational perspectives in clinical practice. Infectious Agents and Cancer. 2017;**12**:36. DOI: 10.1186/ s13027-017-0145-6

[58] Derakhshan Z, Ferrante M, Tadi M, Ansari F, Heydari A, Hosseini MS, et al. Antioxidant activity and total phenolic content of ethanolic extract of pomegranate peels, juice and seeds. Food and Chemical Toxicology. 2018;**114**: 108-111. DOI: 10.1016/j.fct.2018.02.023

[59] AlMatar M, Islam MR, Albarri O, Var I, Koksal F. Pomegranate as a possible treatment in reducing risk of developing wound healing, obesity, neurodegenerative disorders, and diabetes mellitus. Mini Reviews in Medicinal Chemistry. 2018;**18**:507-526. DOI: 10.2174/ 1389557517666170419114722

[60] Caruana M, Cauchi R, Vassallo N. Putative role of red wine polyphenols against brain pathology in Alzheimer's and Parkinson's disease. Frontiers in Nutrition. 2016;**12**(3):31. DOI: 10.3389/ fnut.2016.00031

[61] Cavallini G, Straniero S, Donati A, Bergamini E. Resveratrol requires red wine polyphenols for optimum antioxidant activity. The Journal of Nutrition, Health & Aging. 2016;**20**:540-545. DOI: 10.1007/ s12603-015-0611-z

[62] Kim SJ, Zhang Z, Saha A, Sarkar C, Zhao Z, Xu Y, et al. Omega-3 and omega-6 fatty acids suppress ER- and oxidative stress in cultured neurons and neuronal progenitor cells from mice lacking PPT1. Neuroscience Letters. 2010;**479**:292-296. DOI: 10.1016/j. neulet.2010.05.083

[63] Cavallini G, Sgarbossa A, Parentini I, Bizzarri R, Donati A, Lenci F, et al. Dolichol: A component of the cellular antioxidant machinery. Lipids. 2016;**51**:477-486. DOI: 10.1007/ s11745-016-4137-x

[64] Masoro EJ. Caloric Restriction: A Key to Understanding and Modulating Aging. 1st ed. Vol. 192. Amsterdam, The Netherlands: Elsevier Science; 2002

[65] Bergamini E, Cavallini G, Donati A, Gori Z. The role of autophagy in ageing: Its essential part in the anti-ageing mechanism of caloric restriction. Annals of the New York Academy of Sciences. 2007;**1114**:69-78. DOI: 10.1196/annals.1396.020

[66] Donati A, Taddei M, Cavallini G, Bergamini E. Stimulation of macroautophagy can rescue older cells from 8-OHdG mtDNA accumulation: A safe and easy way to meet goals in the SENS agenda. Rejuvenation Research. 2006;**9**:408-412. DOI: 10.1089/ rej.2006.9.408

[67] Cavallini G, Donati A, Taddei M, Bergamini E. Peroxisomes proliferation and pharmacological stimulation of autophagy in rat liver: Evidence to support that autophagy may remove the "older" peroxisomes. Molecular and Cellular Biochemistry. 2017;**431**:97-102. DOI: 10.1007/ s11010-017-2979-z

[68] Cavallini G, Donati A, Capasso B, Fella M, Leone V, Pezzella G, et al. Effects of stimulation of autophagy on the urinary excretion of biomarkers of the oxidative status. Aging Clinical and Experimental Research. 2014;**26**:13-18. DOI: 10.1007/s40520-013-0116-8

[69] Cathcart R, Schwiers E, Ames BN. Detection of picomole levels of hydroperoxides using a fluorescent dichlorofluorescein assay. Analytical Biochemistry. 1983;**134**:111-116. DOI: 10.1016/0003-2697(83)90270-1

[70] Sharma MK, Buettner GR. Interaction of vitamin C and vitamin E during free radical stress in plasma: An ESR study. Free Radical Biology & Medicine. 1993;**14**:649-653. DOI: 10.1016/0891-5849(93)90146-L

Chapter 4

Long-Term Partnerships in Lewy Body Dementias

Sabina Vatter and Iracema Leroi

Abstract

Long-term partnerships are important as they can determine happiness, influence physical and mental health and lengthen one's lifespan. However, complex neurodegenerative conditions, such as Parkinson's disease dementia (PDD) and dementia with Lewy bodies (DLB), can disrupt long-term relationships and even lead to dissolution of the partnership. The majority of studies in this field have focused on exploring the effect of PDD and DLB on care partners' outcomes but the impact of these conditions on dyadic, long term relationships is less well understood. We conducted a series of studies with people with PDD or DLB and their caregiving life partners using quantitative and qualitative methods. We demonstrated that PDD and DLB has a tremendous impact on the caregiving life partners and reduces relationship satisfaction. We argue for more studies in this field and recommend that future research focuses on strengthening dyadic relationships, which can ultimately preserve relationships and delay institutionalisation of the person with PDD and DLB, which has cost saving implications.

Keywords: long-term relationships, Parkinson's disease dementia, dementia with Lewy bodies, spouse, carer, caregiver, stress-appraisal model

1. Introduction

The prevalence of neurodegenerative conditions, such as Parkinson's disease (PD), Alzheimer's disease (AD) and dementia with Lewy Bodies (DLB) is rapidly growing due to an ageing population. Of the people living with PD, the majority will develop cognitive impairment (PD-MCI) or dementia (PDD) within 20 years of their PD diagnosis. This has implications for the person with the condition, their care partner as well as the wider health and social care economy. Cognitive impairment and dementia are key factors contributing to increases in health care costs, admission to care homes and early mortality. Importantly, these costs can be significantly reduced by the care provided by an informal care partner, usually a family member or a spouse. Such informal care accounts for over £11.6 billion in the United Kingdom (UK) per year [1]. Care partners support the person with a neurodegenerative condition with managing their daily activities as well as their physical and neuropsychiatric symptoms; however, this can impact their mental, emotional, social, financial and physical health.

In this chapter we will examine the nature of the care relationship of long-term partners of people with PDD or DLB, including a theoretical basis for this relationship. We will also outline the impact of the care role with a focus on care burden, quality of life and relationship satisfaction. A deeper understanding of the complex issues surrounding long term care relationships in neurodegenerative conditions such as PDD and DLB is essential in ensuring appropriate support can be put in place.

2. Lewy body dementias (LBD)

PD is a complex progressive neurodegenerative disorder characterised by multiple motor and non-motor symptoms. It affects about 10 million people worldwide and is the second most common neurodegenerative condition after AD [2]. A recent 'Global Burden of Disease Study' found that PD is one of the most rapidly growing neurological conditions for which the number of deaths, prevalent cases and disability-adjusted life years have doubled between 1990 and 2015 [3]. As a result, PD has now been termed 'The Parkinson Pandemic' [4].

While the primary clinical presentation of PD includes a number of motor symptoms including slowness of movement (i.e. bradykinesia), muscular rigidity, rest tremor, or postural instability, a variety of other 'non-motor' symptoms may also manifest. Predominant among these is cognitive impairment and other neuropsychiatric symptoms such as apathy and psychosis which can often be precursors to the onset of PDD [5].

In contrast to PDD, DLB initially presents with cognitive and behavioural symptoms and motor symptoms may not emerge until later in the course of the condition, or in some cases, not at all. PDD and DLB are jointly referred to as 'Lewy body spectrum disorders' [6, 7] or 'Lewy body dementia' (LBD), which is the term we use in this chapter.

2.1 Dementia in PD (PDD)

Dementia in PD (PDD) has become increasingly prevalent with nearly 80% of people with PD developing dementia within 20 years after receiving the diagnosis of PD [8]. PDD is characterised by deterioration in memory, attention, visuospatial functions, executive functions and occurrence of behavioural and psychiatric symptoms, such as apathy and hallucinations [9]. Low cognitive reserve, mild cognitive impairment at baseline, hallucinations and older age, and older age at onset, and the akinetic-rigid motor phenotype are among the main risk factors for developing PDD [9–11].

2.2 Dementia with Lewy bodies (DLB)

DLB is the second most common type of neurodegenerative dementia following AD with a prevalence of 5% of all dementia cases [12]. Pathologically, the distinctive feature of DLB is the appearance of the thread-like protein deposits containing pathologic alpha-synuclein (known as the Lewy bodies) which occur in the central, peripheral, and autonomic nervous system [13]. Symptoms of DLB include cognitive impairment (especially in visuospatial domains and executive function), fluctuating confusion, parkinsonism, visual hallucinations, sleep disturbances and apathy [14]. Recent evidence suggests that 'pure DLB' is less common than 'DLB with concurrent Alzheimer's pathology' due to the overlap of Lewy bodies and neurofibrillary tangles specific to AD [15]. However, cognitive decline is generally faster in DLB than in AD [16] supporting the notion that DLB is an independent disease entity. In 2017, the international clinical diagnostic criteria for DLB were updated and now include guidelines for differentiating between clinical features and diagnostic biomarkers [14].

2.3 Comparison of PDD and DLB

Although PDD and DLB are generally considered part of the same disease spectrum, the initial clinical presentation may differ, due to the timing of the onset of cognitive impairment. However, this view has been challenged [17] and some scholars have concluded that PDD and DLB do not differ with regards to cognitive and neuropsychiatric profile, sleep and autonomic dysfunction, PD type and severity, neuroleptic sensitivity, and responsivity to cholinesterase inhibitors [18–22]. Nonetheless, further studies have demonstrated that significant differences exist between PDD and DLB such as in age of onset (PDD < DLB) [23], levodopa responsiveness (DLB < PDD) [24], neuropsychological test performance (DLB < PDD) [25], and neuropsychiatric presentation [26]. This supports the notion that PDD and DLB are separate clinical conditions but share a common underlying pathology and a distinction should be made on diagnosis.

3. Wider impact of LBD

Both PD and LBD have a significant impact on the person with the condition, their life partner, and family, as well as on society, due to higher needs and dependency as a result of developing the illness. For the person with the condition, the progression of PD can worsen their health-related quality [27], particularly physical and social functioning, cognition, communication and emotional well-being [28]. The notion of adverse impact of PD on physical, social and role functioning is corroborated by a qualitative study which found that PD brings about many changes in emotions and feelings, including fears and uncertainty about the future but also highlights some benefits that PD may bring [29]. Despite the well-established association between subjective well-being and motor impairment, there is a growing literature suggesting that more emphasis should be paid to the positive aspects of well-being, specifically endorsing social support, socialising with other people with PD, engaging in physical activities and maintaining motor skills can contribute to life satisfaction, sense of accomplishment, autonomy and positive emotions in people with PD [27]. This suggests that future studies could focus on life satisfaction and psychological well-being, which could potentially diminish the negative impact of PD on the person.

In terms of the wider impact of PD on society, the disease places a major socioeconomic burden with an estimated annual cost of £2 billion in the UK [30]. A recent report on the impact of living with PD revealed that the total financial costs per household exceeded £16,000 per year due to increase in health and social care costs and reduction in income [31]. Many care partners of people with PD also had to give up employment to be able to provide care for their partner, which led to loss of income [32]. As the severity of PD increases, the costs also rise and can be up to six times higher at the advanced stage (i.e. H&Y stage 5) compared to the initial stage (H&Y stage 1) [33]. These costs likely increase with disease progression due to the complexity of concomitant symptoms of PD, the increasing need for a care partner, and increased rate of admission to residential care homes. However, some of the costs could be partially saved by the help, care and support that family care partners provide to people with PD and LBD. Prince and colleagues [1] estimated that care providers save about £11.6 billion in the UK each year, which is increasing faster than the corresponding increase in formal health and social care costs [1].

Cognitive impairment in PD significantly increases the frequency of institutionalisation [34, 35] and increases healthcare costs even more than PD without cognitive impairment [36, 37]. Furthermore, mortality, which is already increased among people with PD compared to the rest of the population [38], increases with the emergence of dementia, which is one of the key predictors of PD-related mortality [36, 37]. The emergence of cognitive impairment can also significantly decrease quality of life of people with PD and increase emotional stress [39].

Similarly to PD and PDD, a diagnosis of DLB can also escalate healthcare costs [7], shorten time to death [7, 40, 41], and accelerate the rate of admission to residential care homes and hospitals [7, 42]. A DLB diagnosis can also lengthen hospital stay and increase hospitalisation costs [43, 44] compared to AD. Mueller et al. [43] explain that this is due to deteriorated physical health and increased neuropsychiatric symptoms in DLB and they conclude that overall people with DLB have a worse prognosis compared to people with AD [15]. Mueller and colleagues [43] estimate that approximately 80,000 people with DLB in the UK will incur over 27,000 hospital admissions, and spend over 300,000 days in hospital that will exceed £35 million in hospitalisation costs in just 1 year, which is higher compared to the equal number of people with AD.

4. Overview of care partners

Around the world, one person in ten is a care partner [45]. In the UK, there are currently 6.5 million people who provide care and each day 6000 people in addition take on the caring role [46]. Of all the care partners in Great Britain, approximately 11% provide care to someone with dementia in a home setting [47]. Financially, the contribution that care partners make exceeds £132 billion per annum, which surpasses the annual budget of the National Health Service (NHS) in England [48], showing that the help and support that care partners provide is invaluable and has cost saving implications for the health and social care system.

A care partner is an individual, usually a spouse or an adult child, who has taken on the responsibility to help, support and assist a family member who cannot take care of themselves, and to assure they are safe and well [49, 50]. Care provision helps the person with the condition to reach the highest possible functioning in their daily life [49]. Often, the care partner of a person with PD supports with personal, psychological and medical care, assisting with mental and physical exercising, maintaining good nutrition, arranging living conditions and helping with housework [32, 51]. Care partners also coordinate, plan and manage care and look for various interventions and treatments that could potentially alleviate the symptoms of the care recipients [49, 52]. Notably, in addition to providing care, a proportion of care partners may be in part-time or full-time employment [53], which raises complex issues around managing their work and care commitments and may diminish their time and energy to provide care. In addition, care partners may also be older adults themselves and have physical and mental health issues which may limit their capabilities to provide care [51]. As a consequence, care partners, particularly within dementia, may have increased negative feelings, depression, diminished well-being, and neglect their own health [54]. Thus, they become 'the invisible or hidden patients' [52].

Caring and caregiving are considered to be different. Namely, caring is the affective component of 'one's commitment to the welfare of another', whereas caregiving is 'the behavioural expression of this commitment' ([50], p. 583). Likewise, caring has been described as the interplay between emotion and action involving endearing feelings such as love as well as activities involving labour [55]. Caregiving, however, has even been named as the 'unexpected career' due to the sudden onset of this role [56].

The shift into taking on care responsibilities may either be gradual or sudden, although in the case of neurodegenerative conditions such as PDD and DLB, this transition usually occurs gradually. The presenting symptoms of PDD and DLB may be so subtle that care partners may not notice a visible change in their responsibilities, even though they may have started to help and support the care recipients. Thus, in early stages of the disease, care partners may not identify themselves as carers and may even dislike being called a 'carer' [57–59]. Instead, many people prefer to be acknowledged as a 'spouse', 'partner' or 'support person' [58], highlighting the importance of endorsing the relationship between the person receiving care and the person providing it.

The involvement of a care partner in the care of their family member is advantageous because they have a unique perspective on the care recipient's condition and thus, can provide a more precise and detailed description of their symptoms [60]. However, the State of Caring 2018 survey in the UK [48] found that 72% of care partners experienced worsening of their mental health and 61% in their physical health due to their caring role. Furthermore, over half of care partners anticipated that both physical and mental health would continue to deteriorate over the coming years, and a third of participants predicted that a decline in their mental and physical health would prevent them from being able to provide care to the care recipients in the future [48]. Brodaty and Donkin [52] contended that including care partners is so imperative that without their help, the quality of life of people with neurodegenerative conditions would drop so much that it would increase admissions to institutional care. However, this comes at the cost of care partners' own quality of life [52] and raises an important question about how to maintain the well-being of both partners when facing a neurodegenerative condition.

5. Theoretical models of dyadic care relationships in PD

To understand the impact of PD factors on care partners and how they affect care partner well-being and the dyadic relationship, a theoretical framework is required. Such a framework also helps to understand the connections between the variables and to determine the direction of predictors. In the context of dementia, a number of multi-component models have been developed evaluating the factors contributing to caregiving-related stressors [61]. The most common care partner stress models in dementia [61] are:

1. the transactional model of stress and coping [62];

2. the two-dimensional model of psychosocial morbidity [63];

3. the stress process and coping model [64]; and

4. the stress process model [50].

These four preceding models take into account the characteristics of each member of the dyad as well as the care recipient's disease symptomatology and care partner's reactions and outcomes. In PD, the Stress Process Model [50] and the PD-specific Stress-Appraisal Model [65] are most applied by scholars. The Stress-Appraisal model [65] has been built on previous similar models [50, 66–69] and has since been developed further following a systematic review which evaluated burden, mental health and quality of life among care partners of people with PD [70]. The proposed adaptations by Greenwell and colleagues [70] are depicted in **Figure 1**.

The adapted PD-specific Stress-Appraisal model [70], which is derived from the Stress-Appraisal model by Goldsworthy and Knowles [65], captures care partners' experiences of care provision in PD (see **Figure 1**) and consists of four main domains [65, 70]:

1. *Stressors*: care partner well-being is affected by the person with PD factors (= primary stressors), such as neuropsychiatric and cognitive symptoms, their quality of life, their ability to perform activities of daily living and functional dependency (but not motor symptoms), which decreases physical health and increases depression in the care partner (= secondary stressors),

2. *Stress appraisals*: how care partners experience the disease can influence whether they make primary appraisals (i.e. seeing the disease as threatening and thus care partner becomes more involved in care provision by providing more hours of care) or 'secondary appraisals' (i.e. increase of burden and potentially developing coping strategies). Greenwell et al. [43] proposed that tertiary appraisals, which are affected by primary and secondary stressors, secondary appraisal and protective factors, also have a role in determining perceived burden and perceived uplifts by care partner, although burden was seen as a secondary appraisal in Goldsworthy and Knowles' [53] model.

3. *Protective factors (or mediators)*: an important predictor of burden is perceived social support, which can promote well-being or protect from negative consequences of stress. In Goldsworthy and Knowles' [53] model, quality of dyadic relationship, frequency of breaks, formal service hours as well as care partner self-esteem were important mediators in the process of care partner stress appraisal. Greenwell and colleagues [43] suggested that other predictors may include care partner personality traits, sense of coherence and self-efficacy, which require further investigation.

4. *Outcomes*: the impact of primary and secondary stressors; primary, secondary and tertiary appraisals, and protective factors have a direct or indirect impact on care partner outcomes, such as determining their quality of life and depression.

The Stress-Appraisal model is useful in understanding the experiences of care partners in the context of PD and can appropriately be applied to PDD and DLB as well.

Although the Stress-Appraisal model is comprehensive, it does not incorporate the dyadic relationship as an important factor in the context of caregiving relationship. Townsend and Franks [71] proposed the *Binding Ties Theory*, which was designed to

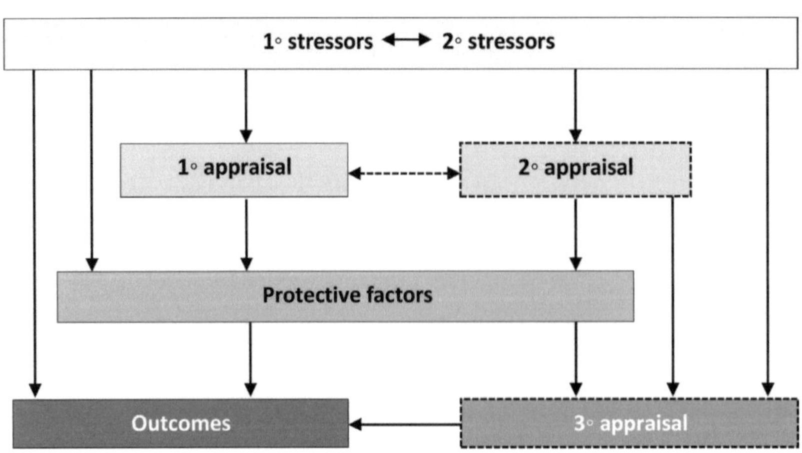

Figure 1.
The stress-appraisal model adapted from Greenwell et al. [70]. The dash line needs further examination. The dash boxes depict alterations to Goldsworthy and Knowles [65] model by Greenwell et al. [70].

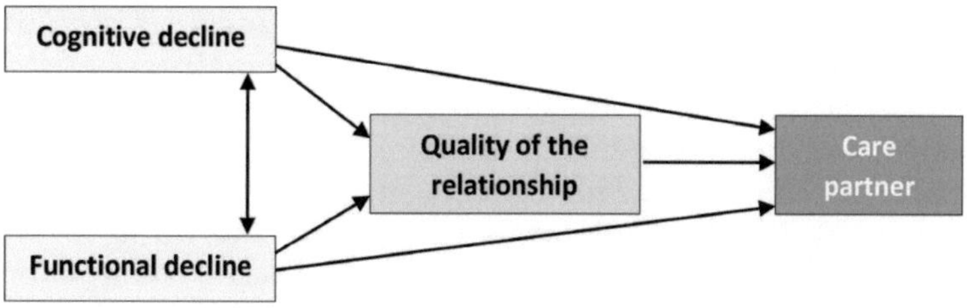

Figure 2.
The binding ties theory [71].

describe the quality of the relationship between adult children and their parents with cognitive impairment (see **Figure 2**). The authors considered the quality of the dyadic relationship to be crucial in care provision and an important determinant in the caregiving experience [71]. The model describes the associations between cognitive and functional impairment, closeness (positive), conflict (negative) and care partner well-being through measures of subjective caregiving stress, subjective caregiving effectiveness and depression. The findings suggest that negative ties were more predictive of care partner well-being than positive ties [71]. Furthermore, the pathway of 'cognitive decline → relationship quality → care partner well-being' was stronger than the 'functional decline → relationship quality → care partner well-being' pathway and advancing cognitive impairment led to less closeness and more conflict in the dyadic relationship [71]. This highlights that studies should evaluate both positive and negative interactions in the context of caregiving relationships.

With regards to the intimate dyadic relationship in PDD and DLB, the Townsend and Franks' [71] model could be incorporated in the Stress-Appraisal model [65, 70] by considering 'cognitive and functional decline' as primary stressors, 'quality of the relationship' as a protective factor and 'care partner well-being' as an outcome.

6. Care provision in LBD

A growing body of research spanning several decades has drawn attention to the impact that LBD has on care partners [70, 72]. The progressive and complex nature of the motor, psychiatric and cognitive symptoms of LBD [73] can reduce one's ability to carry out everyday activities and take care of oneself, thus increasing the need of a care partner. Care partners have a substantial role to play in the lives of people with PDD or DLB as they support and assist with activities of daily living, personal care, medication, feeding, housework, attending specialists' appointments, maintenance of the person's quality of life and independence, and being there as a partner and friend [51, 60, 74, 75]. Commonly, a care partner of a person with PD is a female spouse, aged around 70 years, living with her partner, having provided care for an average of 5 years and currently providing up to 16 hours of care per day [33, 76–79]. Although these descriptions are comparable to those providing care to someone with dementia, the care provision hours in dementia are notably lower than in PD (i.e. 6–9 hours per day) [52].

A recent qualitative meta-synthesis summarised the experiences of PD care partners into four interrelated themes describing (1) the need to carry on as usual, (2) the importance of support in facilitating coping, (3) the difficult balancing act between caregiving and caregiver needs, and (4) conflicts in seeking information and knowledge [80]. Thus, care provision within PD has been considered unique and complex in comparison to other neurodegenerative conditions but to date, little is known about the profile of care partners of people with PDD or DLB.

Studies have evaluated which aspects of PD (in the absence of cognitive impairment) have the highest impact on care partners. Findings suggest that both motor and non-motor symptoms of PD affect care partners' well-being, quality of life and burden but non-motor domains, particularly psychiatric manifestations such as apathy, psychosis, depression and cognitive impairment, tend to have a stronger effect [70, 72, 78, 81–85]. Similarly, the notion that caring for someone with mental illness is emotionally harder, more complex and taxing, as opposed to caring for someone with a physical illness, has been previously posited. This may be due to the changeable, unstable and erratic symptom presentation in mental health conditions, which disrupts 'the coherence of everyday life' ([86], p. 7). This is in line with literature on care partners of people with dementia [52, 87], PD [39, 70] and DLB [74], confirming the complexity of non-motor symptoms in PDD and DLB.

Providing care to a person with PD can be emotionally draining, physically challenging and mentally exhausting for care partners [75, 88]. The impact of PD on care partners is multifaceted, including social, financial, physical, emotional, mental and cognitive aspects. Socially, care partners of people with PD may not be able to go out as much as before, struggle to get away on holidays and have fewer social interactions with their friends, family and neighbours [74, 89–91]. In addition, due to care provision many care partners may be unable to do their usual daily tasks, activities and hobbies, and may receive insufficient social support from friends and family. Having hobbies, being socially active and receiving social support are important because they could protect against worsening of health and well-being [66, 70, 92]. Physically, care partners may experience deterioration in health [90], health-related quality of life [5, 93, 94] and greater fatigue [79].

In terms of mental–emotional aspects, care partners may encounter negative feelings, such as frustration, sadness, anger, resentment, guilt, worry [75, 95], and feel overwhelmed, stressed, strained and burdened [72, 74, 77, 78, 83, 84, 92, 96–98]. Care provision may significantly increase anxiety and depression [89, 93, 95] and lower care partners' mental health [93]. As a consequence, PD care partners' life satisfaction may reduce [95]. Furthermore, in non-PD care partners, the rates of mortality [98], cognitive impairment [99] and relationship dissatisfaction [100] may increase. All of these factors can be escalated with the progression of cognitive impairment in PD [101], which suggests that focusing on the care partners of people with LBD is crucial.

6.1 Physical and mental health

Several studies have found that care provision within PD can worsen mental health and result in distress in care partners [89, 93, 95] compared to the general population. Nearly 50% of care partners of people with PD may experience clinically significant anxiety and depression [72]. Among PD care partners, over a third experienced a deterioration of their health due to care provision [85]. Lack of sleep, fatigue, high blood pressure, muscle strain, headaches and gastrointestinal problems were also common in this group [77] and likely a direct result of providing care. Poor mental health in care partners is directly linked to duration of care provision in years and proportion of hours devoted to caring each day [79]. Moreover, lower levels of mental health are also predicted by care recipients' motor, psychiatric and cognitive symptoms, although drawing definite conclusions about what predicts mental health remains difficult due to the variability of the measures, inconsistent findings and lack of evidence [70]. Importantly, despite the care partners' own health needs, they felt they had to stay healthy as long as possible to be able to care for and support the care recipients [75, 92]. This presents major physical, financial, emotional, mental and social challenges for care partners to continue in their role whilst taking care of themselves.

6.2 Quality of life

Providing care to a person with PD can have a direct effect on care partners' well-being and quality of life. In the literature, quality of life has been synonymously used with other terms such as health, health status, perceived health, functional status, and health-related quality of life although these terms are independent of one another [102]. The concepts of quality of life are wide incorporating economic, environmental, cultural, social, spiritual and personal aspects [103, 104], whereas health-related quality of life specifically focuses on individual's physical, mental and social aspects and the perceptions of their global health [103, 104]. Health-related quality of life has been found to be lower among care partners of people with PD compared to general population [92] and decreases with the emergence and development of cognitive impairment in PD [5, 105, 106].

Quality of life is associated with several factors. Lower quality of life in care partners was predicted by the care recipients' disease-related factors (i.e. motor, cognitive and neuropsychiatric symptom severity, poorer quality of life, higher need for care, greater dependency in activities of daily living), personal aspects (i.e. higher age, depression) and care-related variables (i.e. longer duration of care provision in years and hours per day) [51, 70, 105, 107]. Well-being of care partners is important because lower strain and 'caregiving load' reduces the risk of institutionalising persons with PD [108], which has long-term implications for the future.

6.3 Care burden

As PD progresses, the cognitive impairment advances leading to higher strain [83], burden [5, 76, 78, 106, 109] and stress [82] in care partners. The main contributors to care partner burden and stress in people with PDD were the person's neuropsychiatric symptoms (i.e. depression, psychotic symptoms) [78, 82] and cognitive decline [5, 76, 109, 110]. Apathy, a common and often under-recognised neuropsychiatric complication of PDD and DLB, is strongly associated with care burden [111], in part due to emotional blunting that is one of the dimensions of the apa0thy syndrome [112].

6.3.1 What exactly is 'care burden': a dimensional perspective

One of the most researched constructs in care partner research is 'caregiver burden' [49]. Several different definitions have been proposed but two interwoven descriptions from the 1980s are used concurrently to this day. George and Gwyther [113], p. 253, define burden as 'the physical, psychological or emotional, social, and financial problems that can be experienced by family members caring for impaired older adults'. The same year, Zarit et al. [87], p. 261, proposed a very similar explanation adding that burden is 'the extent to which caregivers perceive their emotional or physical health, social life, and financial status as suffering as a result of caring for their relative'. Even though both explanations encompass the multifaceted impact on care partners, the definitions of burden are still diverse, incoherent and vague in many research studies making measuring 'burden' ambiguous [102, 114]. The authors recommend that burden should be defined clearly, researched using mixed methods (i.e. both quantitatively and qualitatively) and evaluated as specific dimensions of burden [102, 114].

In PD, several different terms exist to refer to burden, for instance *strain* [77, 96, 115, 116], *stress* [117] and *distress* [96, 118]. Despite the fact that these terms have been used instead of burden or in conjunction with burden [84], recent studies have determined that these constructs are independent from burden and are evaluated as separate constructs [72, 76, 84, 119].

One of the most frequently used validated measures of care partner burden is the ZBI [87] which considers 'burden' as a unitary concept. However, burden is highly complex and most likely comprises several dimensions, which have been explored in DLB [120] but not in PDD and DLB jointly. Thus, we undertook a study to explore the factor structure of the ZBI, specifically in life partners of people with PDD or DLB, and to examine the relationships among the emerging factors and the demographic and clinical features in this sample.

In this study [121], we undertook an exploratory factor analysis of the ZBI (principal axis factoring) with 127 life partners. This revealed five burden dimensions: social and psychological constraints, personal strain, interference with personal life, concerns about future, and guilt. These burden factors were associated with lower relationship satisfaction, mental health, and resilience, and higher stress, anxiety, depression, resentment, negative strain and people with PDD/DLB motor severity. In multiple linear regression analyses, where each factor score was the dependent variable, stress, negative strain and resentment emerged as significant predictors of specific burden dimensions. We concluded that burden in PDD and DLB, like in PD in general, is a complex and multidimensional construct and interventions supporting care partners should address specific types of burden to optimise outcomes such as quality of life.

6.3.2 What exactly is 'care burden: life partners' perspectives

To fully explore the meaning of 'care burden' experienced by life partners in the context of PDD and DLB, it is important to go beyond quantitative ratings of burden with typical rating scales such as the ZBI. To address this, we undertook a qualitative study of 12 female life partners of people with PDD and DLB to understand more fully how relationships change as cognition declines in PD [122].

In this study, we undertook semi-structured interviews using a face-to-face format and analysed the outputs using the thematic analysis approach. Our analysis revealed three important, and interlinked, themes: changes in the marital relationship, challenges in providing care, and acceptance and adjustment of the situation, which are discussed below. This study has provided key insights into the changes in long-term marital relationships as dementia progresses in Parkinson's disease.

The theme of 'altered relationship' revealed that the female life partners felt that their relationship satisfaction had decreased as a result of progression in their partners' condition. This was closely linked with partners' reduced ability to communicate and the transition in role for the life partners. Alongside reduced relationship satisfaction, global intimacy as well as emotional, social, recreational, intellectual, physical and sexual intimacies had altered and resulted in life partners feeling emotionally distanced from their partner despite spending more time together. The notion of being physically closer but feeling emotionally further away from their partner was recognised by most life partners in the interviews. This 'emotional disconnection' has been described in the field of dementia [123], as well as the term 'married widowhood' [124, 125]; however, the 'physical closeness' due to day-to-day management of the condition was a finding that emerged in this study, which illustrated the unique challenges that LBD poses in this population.

The second theme, 'care partner challenges' emerged from the complex nature of the motor and non-motor symptoms of LBD as care recipients had lost skills and abilities to do things they were once capable of doing, which in turn increased life partners' responsibilities. Some life partners described they had a dual role in the marriage by being both the man and the woman in the relationship and managing the household, finances, maintenance, car which used to be their spouses' duty. These findings are consistent with previous studies with life partners of people with dementia where life partners took on additional responsibilities while providing care to their partners [123, 126–128]. The increase of care-related responsibilities due to the care recipients' condition was accompanied with an increase in negative feelings and took its toll on life partners. In particular, the time, freedom and independence of wives had reduced to the point of 'losing own life' and becoming mentally and physically weary. As a result of regular care provision, support and surveillance to their partners, wives felt a myriad of feelings such as resentment, frustration, annoyance, sadness, grief, despair, disappointment, guilt, distress and worry.

Finally, the third theme to emerge, 'acceptance and adjustment', captured life partners' acceptance of care provision as part of their marital contract and saw it inseparable from their commitments to the relationship with their partner. In spite of the challenges, difficulties and negative feelings that wives experienced and confronted with due to providing care, they revealed feelings of love, compassion, empathy and sympathy towards their partner. People with DLB had cared for their wives throughout their married life when they needed help due to health ailments and this reciprocity was acknowledged by life partners who felt they had to reciprocate the care for as long as they could. Life partners in this study and in other qualitative studies were committed to their marital vows and held onto the 'in sickness and in health, till death do us apart' but there was also some confusion whether the marriage still existed as dementia progressed [129–132]. Notwithstanding the conflict between existence and loss of relationship, life partners felt committed to their partners and were willing to continue providing care to their spouse in the future.

6.4 The influence of LBD on care partner outcomes

Comparative studies between care partners of people with different neurodegenerative conditions have shown important distinctions. In one study, burden in care partners was higher in PDD compared to AD, with neuropsychiatric disturbances fundamentally contributing to burden in care partners of people with PDD [133]. Another study supported these findings and added that care partners of people with PDD experienced more depression, lower satisfaction with life and needed more help and assistance compared to care partners of people with PD and AD [101]. Similarly, care partners of people with DLB had higher burden [134] and distress [135, 136] compared to care partners of people with AD and frontotemporal lobar degeneration [137] due to more prominent neuropsychiatric symptoms in DLB. Care partners of both people with PDD and DLB also experienced higher levels of stress compared to AD and vascular dementia [138]. To examine this issue further, we undertook a study comparing the characteristics of care partners in three groups of people with different clinical profiles of Parkinson's-related cognitive impairment: PD-MCI, PDD and DLB.

6.4.1 Study of care partner characteristics in LBD

In our study [139] we aimed to describe the sociodemographic and clinical profile of life partners of people with different cognitive syndromes in LBD, including physical and mental health, burden, stress, quality of life and feelings related to care provision, and compare life partners' outcomes according to the clinical syndrome (PD-MCI, PDD or DLB). The study involved a cross-sectional assessment battery undertaken by 136 co-resident life partners who completed ratings of overall mental well-being, anxiety, depression, burden, stress and aspects of the relationship such as satisfaction. We found that the majority of participants were women (85%), with a mean age of 69 years (SD = 7.62; range 48–85 years) who had been in an intimate relationship for a median of 45 years. Life partners had provided care for between 0 and 20 years (median = 4; IQR = 2–7) and at the time of the study, were currently providing care between 0 and 168 hours per week (median = 84; IQR = 38.5–168). Nearly half of the participants (46.0%) provided over 100 hours of care per week.

Our assessments revealed that over 25% of the life partners were experiencing clinically significant anxiety and over 10% were experiencing significant depression, as per cut-off scores on the Hospital Anxiety and Depression Scale [140]. Findings on the Relatives' Stress scale [141] and the Zarit Burden Interview (ZBI) [87] revealed that nearly 60% of participants were experiencing significant stress and over 30% were experiencing significant burden. About 60% of life partners reported dissatisfaction with the relationship, as determined by the Relationship Satisfaction Scale [142] and slightly fewer than half reported quality of life that was lower than 'good', as per the EQ-5D index scores and visual analogue scale [143]. Overall, the majority of caregiving life partners reported satisfaction with their caring role; however, over 60% of life partners displayed resentment (63%) and over 30% anger in relation to this role (measured with the Family Caregiving Role Scale, [144]).

These findings of high levels of burden, stress and feelings of resentment and anger among life partners resonated with earlier findings of high levels of stress, burden and quality of life among care partners of people with PD, PDD, and DLB [5, 39, 72, 78, 145]. However, relationship dissatisfaction, perceived negative feelings, such as resentment, and resilience are new findings emerging from this study and appear to be under-researched in the field of LBD, despite numerous studies evaluating these constructs in other types of dementia [129, 146, 147]. This is important as it could be hypothesised that care partner outcomes could be similar in LBD and other types of dementia, but evidence suggests that rates of burden, stress, depression, as well as physical health outcomes are worse in partners of people with PDD and DLB compared to other forms of dementia [101, 133, 134, 136, 138]. Furthermore, tensions and arguments in the dyadic relationship [126] and lower abilities to live well [148] appear in PDD and DLB care partners, compared to care partners of people with AD and/or vascular dementia. This suggests that care partners of people with PDD or DLB may require more support. Importantly, our finding that care provision by over half of life partners exceeded 14 hours each day and over 100 hours each week, which is significantly higher compared to the rest of care partners in the UK [149], emphasised the complexity of providing care for a person with PDD or DLB as well as the immense commitment by life partners in providing the care.

Furthermore, we found that characteristics of life partners differed according to the clinical profile of the care recipient [139]. As expected, life partners of people with PDD had provided care for more years than life partners of people with PD-MCI, and life partners of people with PDD and DLB were providing more hours of care each week than life partners of people with PD-MCI. A linear relationship was found between several variables and progression of cognitive impairment in PD. Once dementia in PD had emerged, life partners were more burdened, stressed, depressed, resentful, dissatisfied with the relationship and experienced fewer positive interactions with their partner compared to those whose partner had PD-MCI. Similarly to PDD, life partners of people with DLB had higher rates of depression, burden and feelings of resentment in comparison to life partners of people with PD-MCI. Importantly, life partners of people with DLB had higher anxiety levels and reported lower levels of mental health compared to life partners of people with PD-MCI, whereas these outcomes did not differ between PD-MCI and PDD groups, suggesting that specific clinical syndrome plays an important role in determining life partner outcomes.

7. Overview of dyadic relationships

Relationship quality is a multifactorial construct and can be broken down into overall satisfaction, commitment, closeness or intimacy, passion, trust and love [150]. Spanier [151], p. 290, defined relationship quality as 'a subjective evaluation of a married couple's relationship with the range of evaluations constituting a continuum reflecting numerous characteristics of marital interaction and marital functioning'. In the context of marriage, relationship quality encompasses adjustment, satisfaction, integration and happiness and can be seen in terms of its functionality and how the partners are affected by its functioning [151].

Relationship satisfaction is one of the key components of relationship quality. It has been defined in the context of interdependence theory [152, 153], which sees the interaction between partners, dependence and satisfaction as the core elements in close intimate relationships [154]. The dyadic *interaction* consists of rewards (i.e. pleasure, enjoyment, fulfilment) as well as costs (i.e. stress, pain, shame) that each partner may receive in the relationship. The goal is to minimise costs and maximise rewards [154]. Relationship satisfaction is affected by the level of one partner fulfilling the most significant needs of the other partner [155]. Each individual assesses the gains and benefits in their relationship as well as outputs they give to their partner. Relationship satisfaction is higher when the input-outcome ratio equates with that of the partner, whereas an imbalance in the ratio leads to dissatisfaction with the relationship [154].

8. Dyadic relationships in LBD

Both dementia and PD have a profound effect on the person, the care partner and their relationship [156]. People with PD have reported significant reduction in sexual functions, although the non-sexual relationship aspects, for example talking about one's feelings or tenderness, increased with the duration of the disease [157]. Men with PD tend to withdraw from the relationship, may have had increased thoughts of divorce and may have reported dissatisfaction with the relationship and sexuality since the onset of PD, more so than women with PD [157]. Mutuality, defined as the positive quality of a partnership consisting of love and affection, reciprocity, shared values and shared pleasurable activities [158], remains relatively high at mild to moderate stages of PD but can be significantly lower at an advanced stage of PD [83, 159]. Likewise, in another study, both partners' mutuality levels were similar but people with PD reported higher reciprocity than their partners [159]. Mutuality, alongside with non-motor symptoms, was also found to be a predictor of health-related quality of life for people with PD, whereas mutuality and cognition were the main predictors of burden in life partners [159]. These studies highlight that the impact of PD on the couple is substantial.

The advancing nature of dementia increases the person's memory loss, confusion, agitation and inability to communicate, which may lead them to not recognising one's partner and forgetting that they are married [129]. As a consequence, the life partner might start to doubt whether the marriage still exists [129]. Thus, the central theme describing relationships within dementia is often 'loss'–loss of a person, relationship, mutual companionship and connectedness [123, 129]. This theme also applies in PD as life partners of people with PD experienced feelings of loss and helplessness and felt overwhelmed and unable to cope with the cognitive impairment of the care recipient [39], highlighting that once cognition has started to decline, the impact is more profound compared to intact PD.

Neurodegenerative conditions, such as PDD and DLB, can challenge a couple and impact negatively on relationship quality and lead to dissatisfaction even more than other diseases due to its incurable and progressive nature. Evidence outside of PD has revealed that one partners' depression can contribute to relationship dissatisfaction, lower levels of communication and problem-solving abilities as well as difficulties maintaining intimacy [160]. In turn, higher loss of intimacy can lead to higher levels of depression [161]. Similarly, lower marital quality in people with PD can contribute to higher anxiety in life partners [162]. In cognitively intact people with PD, the motor symptoms had a significant impact on the relationship [163] but when cognitive decline had emerged, non-motor symptoms were the most prominent stressors on couples' relationships [159]. In order to overcome the challenges and sustain relationships, efficient and effective coping strategies are required. Lack of these strategies can lead to increased burden and health issues in the care partner, institutionalisation of the person with LBD and eventually relationship breakdown [164].

Importantly, having a close relationship with one's partner can be protective. More satisfaction with intimacy was associated with less stress and fewer depressive symptoms, particularly in female care partners [165]. In PD, higher mutuality was related to better mental health outcomes for partners, lower PD severity as well as lower burden and higher quality of life in the care partner [163]. The ability to remain positive when having PD or living with a care recipient who has PD has been found to contribute to higher marital quality for the couple [162]. These findings resonate with Habermann's [166] study who stated that PD affected couples' closeness and communication positively. Despite these encouraging findings, PD has been found to have a detrimental effect on the relationship and lead to poor marital adjustment [167]. Thus, further research is required to explore the consequences of PD and LBD on the person, life partner and their relationship.

9. Conclusion

This chapter has highlighted the profound impact of LBD on life partners, in particular due to psychiatric and cognitive symptoms of people with PDD and DLB which intensify with the progression of cognitive impairment in PD. As a result of providing care to people with LBD, life partners experience burden, stress, poor mental health, negative feelings and relationship dissatisfaction, and for many life partners their life had changed as a result of becoming a care partner. There is currently minimal targeted support available to couples within LBD but in light of the protective nature of good relationships, future studies should focus on supporting intimate relationships resulting in more positive outcomes for both partners.

Conflict of interest

The authors have no financial conflicts.
This chapter is based on a doctoral thesis [168].

Author details

Sabina Vatter[1] and Iracema Leroi[1,2]*

1 Faculty of Biology, Medicine and Health, Division of Neuroscience and Experimental Psychology, School of Biological Sciences, University of Manchester, United Kingdom

2 Global Brain Health Institute, Trinity College Dublin, Ireland

*Address all correspondence to: iracema.leroi@tcd.ie

References

[1] Prince M, Knapp M, Guerchet M, et al. Dementia UK: Second Edition—Overview. London, UK: Alzheimer's Society; 2014

[2] European Parkinson's Disease Association [EPDA]. What is Parkinson's? 2018. Abvailable from: www.epda.eu.com/about-parkinsons/what-is-parkinsons [Accessed: January 31, 2019]

[3] GBD 2015 Neurological Disorders Collaborator Group. Global, regional, and national burden of neurological disorders during 1990-2015: A systematic analysis for the Global Burden of Disease Study 2015. Lancet Neurology. 2017;**16**:877-897

[4] Dorsey ER, Bloem BR. The Parkinson pandemic—A call to action. JAMA Neurology. 2018;75:9-10

[5] Leroi I, McDonald K, Pantula H, Harbishettar V. Cognitive impairment in Parkinson disease: Impact on quality of life, disability, and caregiver burden. Journal of Geriatric Psychiatry and Neurology. 2012;**25**:208-214

[6] Goldman JG, Williams-Gray C, Barker RA, et al. The spectrum of cognitive impairment in Lewy body diseases. Movement Disorders. 2014;**29**:608-621

[7] Zweig YR, Galvin JE. Lewy body dementia: The impact on patients and caregivers. Alzheimer's Research and Therapy. 2014;**6**:21

[8] Hely MA, Reid WG, Adena MA, et al. The Sydney multicenter study of Parkinson's disease: The inevitability of dementia at 20 years. Movement Disorders. 2008;**23**:837-844

[9] Emre M, Aarsland D, Brown R, et al. Clinical diagnostic criteria for dementia associated with Parkinson's disease. Movement Disorders. 2007;**22**:1689-1707

[10] Aarsland D, Andersen K, Larsen JP, et al. Prevalence and characteristics of dementia in Parkinson disease: An 8-year prospective study. Archives of Neurology. 2003;**60**:387-392

[11] Riedel O, Klotsche J, Spottke A, et al. Cognitive impairment in 873 patients with idiopathic Parkinson's disease. Results from the German study on epidemiology of Parkinson's disease with dementia (GEPAD). Journal of Neurology. 2008;**255**:255-264

[12] Kane JPM, Surendranathan A, Bentley A, et al. Clinical prevalence of Lewy body dementia. Alzheimer's Research and Therapy. 2018;**10**:19

[13] Jellinger KA. Formation and development of Lewy pathology: A critical update. Journal of Neurology. 2009;**256**:270-279

[14] McKeith IG, Boeve BF, Dickson DW, et al. Diagnosis and management of dementia with Lewy bodies: Fourth consensus report of the DLB consortium. Neurology. 2017;**89**:88-100

[15] Mueller C, Ballard C, Corbett A, Aarsland D. The prognosis of dementia with Lewy bodies. Lancet Neurology. 2017;**16**:390-398

[16] Rongve A, Soennesyn H, Skogseth R, et al. Cognitive decline in dementia with Lewy bodies: A 5-year prospective cohort study. BMJ Open. 2016;**6**:e010357

[17] Taylor JP, O'Brien JT. Parkinson's disease with dementia. In: Ebmeier KP, O'Brien JT, Taylor JP, editors. Psychiatry of Parkinson's Disease. Advances in Biological Psychiatry. Basel: Karger; 2012. pp. 103-124

[18] Aldridge GM, Birnschein A, Denburg NL, Narayanan NS. Parkinson's disease dementia and dementia with Lewy bodies have similar

neuropsychological profiles. Frontiers in Neurology. 2018;**9**:123

[19] Friedman JH. Dementia with Lewy bodies and Parkinson disease dementia: It is the same disease! Parkinsonism and Related Disorders. 2018;**46**:S6-S9

[20] Jellinger KA, Korczyn AD. Are dementia with Lewy bodies and Parkinson's disease dementia the same disease? BMC Medicine. 2018;**16**:34

[21] McKeith IG, Mintzer J, Aarsland D, et al. Dementia with Lewy bodies. Lancet Neurology. 2014;**3**:19-28

[22] McShane R. Clinical aspects of dementia: Dementia in Parkinson's disease and dementia with Lewy bodies. In: Jacoby R, Oppenheimer C, Dening T, Thomas A, editors. Old Age Psychiatry. 4th ed. New York: Oxford University Press; 2008. pp. 453-459

[23] Fields JA. Cognitive and neuropsychiatric features in Parkinson's and Lewy body dementias. Archives of Clinical Neuropsychology. 2017;**32**:786-801

[24] Dodel R, Csoti I, Ebersbach G, et al. Lewy body dementia and Parkinson's disease with dementia. Journal of Neurology. 2008;**255**:39-47

[25] Mondon K, Gochard A, Marque A, et al. Visual recognition memory differentiates dementia with Lewy bodies and Parkinson's disease dementia. Journal of Neurology, Neurosurgery and Psychiatry. 2007;**78**:738-741

[26] Chiu PY, Tsai CT, Chen PK, et al. Neuropsychiatric symptoms in Parkinson's disease dementia are more similar to Alzheimer's disease than dementia with Lewy bodies: A case-control study. PLoS One. 2016;**11**:e0153989

[27] Vescovelli F, Sarti D, Ruini C. Subjective and psychological well-being in Parkinson's disease: A systematic review. Acta Neurologica Scandinavica. 2018;**138**:12-23

[28] Schrag A, Jahanshahi M Quinn N. What contributes to quality of life in patients with Parkinson's disease? Journal of Neurology. Neurosurgery and Psychiatry. 2000;**69**:308-312

[29] Chiong-Rivero H, Ryan GW, Flippen C, et al. Patients' and caregivers' experiences of the impact of Parkinson's disease on health status. Patient Related Outcome Measures. 2011;**2**:57-70

[30] Wong S. Imperial College London. Cost of Brain Disorders to the UK Estimated at £112 Billion a Year. 2013. Available from: www.imperial.ac.uk/news/126466/cost-brain-disorders-uk-estimated-112 [Accessed: February 5, 2019]

[31] Gumber A, Ramaswamy B, Ibbotson R, et al. Economic, social and financial cost of Parkinson's on individuals, carers and their families in the UK. Sheffield, UK: Centre for Health and Social Care Research, Sheffield Hallam University; 2017

[32] McLaughlin D, Hasson F, Kernohan WG, et al. Living and coping with Parkinson's disease: Perceptions of informal carers. Palliative Medicine. 2010;**25**:177-182

[33] Findley LJ. The economic impact of Parkinson's disease. Parkinsonism and Related Disorders. 2007;**13**:S8-S12

[34] Aarsland D, Larsen JP, Tandberg E, Laake K. Predictors of nursing home placement in Parkinson's disease: A population-based, prospective study. Journal of the American Geriatrics Society. 2000;**48**:938-942

[35] Safarpour D, Thibault DP, DeSanto CL, et al. Nursing home and end-of-life care in Parkinson disease. Neurology. 2015;**85**:413-419

[36] Hughes TA, Ross HF, Mindham RH, Spokes EG. Mortality in Parkinson's disease and its association with dementia and depression. Acta Neurologica Scandinavica. 2004;**110**:118-123

[37] Larsson V, Torisson G, Londos E. Relative survival in patients with dementia with Lewy bodies and Parkinson's disease dementia. PLoS One. 2018;**13**:e0202044

[38] Hobson P, Meara J. Mild cognitive impairment in Parkinson's disease and its progression onto dementia: A 16-year outcome evaluation of the Denbighshire cohort. International Journal of Geriatric Psychiatry. 2015;**30**:1048-1055

[39] Lawson RA, Collerton D, Taylor JP, et al. Coping with cognitive impairment in people with Parkinson's disease and their carers: A qualitative study. Parkinson's disease. 2018:1362053

[40] Oesterhus R, Soennesyn H, Rongve A, et al. Long-term mortality in a cohort of home-dwelling elderly with mild Alzheimer's disease and Lewy body dementia. Dementia and Geriatric Cognitive Disorders. 2014;**38**:161-169

[41] Price A, Farooq R, Yuan JM, et al. Mortality in dementia with Lewy bodies compared with Alzheimer's dementia: A retrospective naturalistic cohort study. BMJ Open. 2017;**7**:e017504

[42] Rongve A, Vossius C, Nore S, et al. Time until nursing home admission in people with mild dementia: Comparison of dementia with Lewy bodies and Alzheimer's dementia. International Journal of Geriatric Psychiatry. 2014;**29**:392-398

[43] Mueller C, Perera G, Rajkumar AP, et al. Hospitalization in people with dementia with Lewy bodies: Frequency, duration, and cost implications. Alzheimer's Dementia: Diagnosis, Assessment and Disease Monitoring. 2018;**10**:143-152

[44] Vossius C, Rongve A, Testad I, et al. The use and costs of formal care in newly diagnosed dementia: A three-year prospective follow-up study. The American Journal of Geriatric Psychiatry. 2014;**22**:381-388

[45] Office for National Statistics [ONS] 2011 Census Data. 2011. Available from: www.ons.gov.uk/census/2011census/2011censusdata [Accessed: February 3, 2019]

[46] Carers UK. Why We're Here. 2014. Available from: www.carersuk.org/about-us/why-we-re-here [Accessed: February 3, 2019]

[47] Carers Trust. Key Facts About Carers and the People They Care for. 2015. Available from: https://carers.org/key-facts-about-carers-and-people-they-care [Accessed: February 3, 2019]

[48] Carers UK. State of Caring 2018 Here. 2018. Available from: www.carersuk.org/images/Downloads/SoC2018/State-of-Caring-report-2018.pdf [Accessed: February 3, 2019]

[49] Ham RJ. Evolving standards in patient and caregiver support. Alzheimer Disease and Associated Disorders. 1999;**13**:S27-S35

[50] Pearlin LI, Mullan JT, Semple SJ, Skaff MM. Caregiving and the stress process: An overview of concepts and their measures. The Gerontologist. 1990;**30**:583-594

[51] Hand A, Oates LL, Gray WK, Walker RW. The role and profile of the informal carer in meeting the needs of people with advancing Parkinson's disease. Aging and Mental Health. 2018;**23**:337-344. DOI: 10.1080/13607863.2017.1421612

[52] Brodaty H, Donkin M. Family caregivers of people with dementia.

Dialogues in Clinical Neuroscience. 2009;**11**:217-228

[53] Ostwald SK. Caregiver exhaustion: Caring for the hidden patients. Advanced Practice Nursing Quarterly. 1997;**3**:29-35

[54] Pinquart M, Sörensen S. Differences between caregivers and noncaregivers in psychological health and physical health: A meta-analysis. Psychology and Aging. 2003;**18**:250-267

[55] Hennings J, Froggatt K, Payne S. Spouse caregivers of people with advanced dementia in nursing homes: A longitudinal narrative study. Palliative Medicine. 2013;**27**:683-691

[56] Pearlin LI, Aneshensel CS. Caregiving: The unexpected career. Social Justice Research. 1994;7:373-390

[57] Gaugler JE, Kane RL, Kane RA. Family care for older adults with disabilities: Toward more targeted and interpretable research. International Journal of Aging and Human Development. 2002;**54**:205-231

[58] Leroi I. Disrupted identities: Movement, mind, and memory in Parkinson's disease. International Psychogeriatrics. 2017;**29**:879-881

[59] Molyneaux VJ, Butchard S, Simpson J, Murray C. The co-construction of couplehood in dementia. Dementia. 2011;**11**(4):483-502

[60] Hiseman JP, Fackrell R. Caregiver burden and the nonmotor symptoms of Parkinson's disease. International Review of Neurobiology. 2017;**133**:479-497

[61] van der Lee J, Bakker TJ, Duivenvoorden HJ, Dröes RM. Multivariate models of subjective caregiver burden in dementia: A systematic review. Ageing Research Reviews. 2014;**15**:76-93

[62] Lazarus RS, Folkman S. Stress, Appraisal, and Coping. New York: Springer Publishing Company; 1984

[63] Poulshock SW, Deimling GT. Families caring for elders in residence: Issues in the measurement of burden. Journal of Gerontology. 1984;**39**:230-239

[64] Haley WE, Levine EG, Brown SL, Bartolucci AA. Stress, appraisal, coping, and social support as predictors of adaptational outcome among dementia caregivers. Psychology and Aging. 1987;**2**:323-330

[65] Goldsworthy B, Knowles S. Caregiving for Parkinson's disease patients: An exploration of a stress-appraisal model for quality of life and burden. The Journals of Gerontology: Series B, Psychological Sciences and Social Sciences. 2008;**63**:P372-P376

[66] Chappell NL, Reid RC. Burden and well-being among caregivers: Examining the distinction. The Gerontologist. 2002;**42**:772-780

[67] Lawton MP, Klcban MH, Moss M, et al. Measuring caregiving appraisal. Journal of Gerontology. 1989;**44**:61-71

[68] Lawton MP, Moss M, Kleban MH, et al. A two-factor model of caregiving appraisal and psychological well-being. Journal of Gerontology. 1991;**46**:181-189

[69] Yates ME, Tennstedt S, Chang BH. Contributors to and mediators of psychological well-being for informal caregivers. The Journals of Gerontology: Series B, Psychological Sciences and Social Sciences. 1999;**54**:P12-P22

[70] Greenwell K, Gray WK, van Wersch A, et al. Predictors of the psychosocial impact of being a carer of people living with Parkinson's disease: A systematic review. Parkinsonism and Related Disorders. 2015;**21**:1-11

[71] Townsend AL, Franks MM. Binding ties: Closeness and conflict in adult children's caregiving relationships. Psychological Aging. 1995;**10**:343-351

[72] Mosley PE, Moodie R, Dissanayaka N. Caregiver burden in Parkinson disease: A critical review of recent literature. Journal of Geriatric Psychiatry and Neurology. 2017;**30**:235-252

[73] Chaudhuri KR, Healy DG, Schapira AHV. Non-motor symptoms of Parkinson's disease: Diagnosis and management. Lancet Neurology. 2006;**5**:235-245

[74] Galvin JE, Duda JE, Kaufer DI, et al. Lewy body dementia: Caregiver burden and unmet needs. Alzheimer Disease and Associated Disorders. 2010;**24**:177-181

[75] Tan SB, Williams AF, Morris ME. Experiences of caregivers of people with Parkinson's disease in Singapore: A qualitative analysis. Journal of Clinical Nursing. 2012;**21**:2235-2246

[76] Cifu DX, Carne W, Brown R, et al. Caregiver distress in parkinsonism. Journal of Rehabilitation Research and Development. 2006;**43**:499-508

[77] Lökk J. Caregiver strain in Parkinson's disease and the impact of disease duration. European Journal of Physical and Rehabilitation Medicine. 2008;**44**:39-45

[78] Martinez-Martin P, Rodriguez-Blazquez C, Forjaz MJ, et al. Neuropsychiatric symptoms and caregiver's burden in Parkinson's disease. Parkinsonism and Related Disorders. 2015;**21**:629-634

[79] Peters M, Fitzpatrick R, Doll H, et al. Does self-reported well-being of patients with Parkinson's disease influence caregiver strain and quality of life? Parkinsonism and Related Disorders. 2011;**17**:348-352

[80] Theed R, Eccles F, Simpson J. Experiences of caring for a family member with Parkinson's disease: A meta-synthesis. Aging and Mental Health. 2017;**21**:1007-1016

[81] Aarsland D, Larsen JP, Lim NG, et al. Range of neuropsychiatric disturbances in patients with Parkinson's disease. Journal of Neurology, Neurosurgery, and Psychiatry. 1999;**67**:492-496

[82] Aarsland D, Brønnick K, Ehrt U, et al. Neuropsychiatric symptoms in patients with Parkinson's disease and dementia: Frequency, profile and associated care giver stress. Journal of Neurology, Neurosurgery, and Psychiatry. 2007;**78**:36-42

[83] Carter JH, Stewart BJ, Lyons KS, Archbold PG. Do motor and nonmotor symptoms in PD patients predict caregiver strain and depression? Movement Disorders. 2008;**23**:1211-1216

[84] Leiknes I, Lien UT, Severinsson E. The relationship among caregiver burden, demographic variables, and the clinical characteristics of patients with Parkinson's disease—A systematic review of studies using various caregiver burden instruments. Open Journal of Nursing. 2015;**5**:855-877

[85] Schrag A, Hovris A, Morley D, et al. Caregiver-burden in Parkinson's disease is closely associated with psychiatric symptoms, falls, and disability. Parkinsonism and Related Disorders. 2006;**12**:35-41

[86] Karp DA, Tanarugsachock V. Mental illness, caregiving, and emotion management. Qualitative Health Research. 2000;**10**:6-25

[87] Zarit SH, Todd PA, Zarit JM. Subjective burden of husbands and

wives as caregivers: A longitudinal study. The Gerontologist. 1986;**26**:260-266

[88] Roland KP, Jenkins ME, Johnson AM. An exploration of the burden experienced by spousal caregivers of individuals with Parkinson's disease. Movement Disorders. 2010;**25**:189-193

[89] Pinquart M, Sörensen S. Correlates of physical health of informal caregivers: A meta-analysis. The Journals of Gerontology: Series B, Psychological Sciences and Social Sciences. 2007;**62**:P126-P137

[90] O'Reilly F, Finnan F, Allwright S, et al. The effects of caring for a spouse with Parkinson's disease on social, psychological and physical well-being. The British Journal of General Practice. 1996;**46**:507-512

[91] Thommessen B, Aarsland D, Braekhus A, et al. The psychosocial burden on spouses of the elderly with stroke, dementia and Parkinson's disease. International Journal of Geriatric Psychiatry. 2002;**17**:78-84

[92] Berger S, Chen T, Eldridge J, et al. The self-management balancing act of spousal care partners in the case of Parkinson's disease. Disability and Rehabilitation. 2017;**41**:887-895. DOI: 10.1080/09638288.2017.1413427

[93] Martinez-Martin P, Arroyo S, Rojo-Abuin JM, et al. Burden, perceived health status, and mood among caregivers of Parkinson's disease patients. Movement Disorders. 2008;**23**:1673-1680

[94] Lawson RA, Yarnall AJ, Johnston F, et al. Cognitive impairment in Parkinson's disease: Impact on quality of life of carers. International Journal of Geriatric Psychiatry. 2017;**32**:1362-1370

[95] Aarsland D, Larsen JP, Karlsen K, et al. Mental symptoms in Parkinson's disease are important contributors to caregiver distress. International Journal of Geriatric Psychiatry. 1999;**14**:866-874

[96] Miller E, Berrios GE, Politynska BE. Caring for someone with Parkinson's disease: Factors that contribute to distress. International Journal of Geriatric Psychiatry. 1996;**11**:263-268

[97] Whetten-Goldstein K, Sloan F, Kulas E, et al. The burden of Parkinson's disease on society, family, and the individual. Journal of the American Geriatrics Society. 1997;**45**:844-849

[98] Schulz R, Beach SR. Caregiving as a risk factor for mortality: The caregiver health effects study. Journal of the American Medical Association. 1999;**282**:2215-2219

[99] Mallya S, Fiocco AJ. Impact of informal caregiving on cognitive function and well-being in Canada. International Psychogeriatrics. 2018;**30**:1049-1055

[100] Steadman PL, Tremont G, Duncan Davis J. Premorbid relationship satisfaction and caregiver burden in dementia caregivers. Journal of Geriatric Psychiatry and Neurology. 2007;**20**:115-119

[101] Roland KP, Chappell NL. Caregiver experiences across three neurodegenerative diseases: Alzheimer's, Parkinson's and Parkinson's with dementia. Journal of Aging and Health. 2019;**31**:256-279. DOI: 10.1177/0898264317729980

[102] Braithwaite V. Caregiving burden: Making the concept scientifically useful and policy relevant. Research on Aging. 1992;**14**:3-27

[103] Martinez-Martin P. What is quality of life and how do we measure it? Relevance to Parkinson's disease and movement disorders. Movement Disorders. 2017;**32**:382-392

[104] World Health Organization [WHO]. WHOQOL: Measuring Quality of Life. Geneva, Switzerland: World Health Organization; 1997

[105] Martinez-Martin P, Benito-Leon J, Alonso F, et al. Quality of life of caregivers in Parkinson's disease. Quality of Life Research. 2005;**14**:463-472

[106] Szeto JY, Mowszowski L, Gilat M, et al. Mild cognitive impairment in Parkinson's disease: Impact on caregiver outcomes. Journal of Parkinson's Disease. 2016;**6**:589-596

[107] Morley D, Dummett S, Peters M, et al. Factors influencing quality of life in caregivers of people with Parkinson's disease and implications for clinical guidelines. Parkinson's Disease. 2012;**190901**:1-6

[108] Abendroth M, Lutz BJ, Young ME. Family caregivers' decision process to institutionalize persons with Parkinson's disease: A grounded theory study. International Journal of Nursing Studies. 2012;**49**:445-454

[109] Jones AJ, Kuijer RG, Livingston L, et al. Caregiver burden is increased in Parkinson's disease with mild cognitive impairment (PD-MCI). Translational Neurodegeneration. 2017;**6**:17

[110] Leroi I, Ahearn DJ, Andrews M, et al. Behavioural disorders, disability and quality of life in Parkinson's disease. Age and Ageing. 2011;**40**:614-621

[111] Leroi I, Harbishettar V, Andrews M, et al. Carer burden in apathy and impulse control disorders in Parkinson's disease. International Journal of Geriatric Psychiatry. 2012;**27**:160-166

[112] Leroi I, Perera N, Harbishettar V, Robert P. Apathy and emotional blunting in Parkinson's disease. Brain Disorders and Therapy. 2014;**3**:141

[113] George LK, Gwyther LP. Caregiver well-being: A multidimensional examination of family caregivers of demented adults. The Gerontologist. 1986;**26**:253-259

[114] Bastawrous M. Caregiver burden—A critical discussion. International Journal of Nursing Studies. 2013;**50**:431-441

[115] Kelly DH, McGinley JL, Huxham FE, et al. Health-related quality of life and strain in caregivers of Australians with Parkinson's disease: An observational study. BMC Neurology. 2012;**12**:57

[116] Nygaard HA. Strain on caregivers of demented elderly people living at home. Scandinavian Journal of Primary Health Care. 1988;**6**:33-37

[117] McRae C, Sherry P, Roper K. Stress and family functioning among caregivers of persons with Parkinson's disease. Parkinsonism and Related Disorders. 1999;**5**:69-75

[118] Lau KM, Au A. Correlates of informal caregiver distress in Parkinson's disease: A meta-analysis. Clinical Gerontologist. 2011;**34**:117-131

[119] Santos-Garcia D, de la Fuente-Fernandez R. Factors contributing to caregivers' stress and burden in Parkinson's disease. Acta Neurologica Scandinavica. 2015;**131**:203-210

[120] Leggett AN, Zarit S, Taylor A, Galvin JE. Stress and burden among caregivers of patients with Lewy body dementia. The Gerontologist. 2011;**51**:76-85

[121] Vatter S, McDonald KR, Stanmore E, et al. Multidimensional care burden in Parkinson-related dementia. Journal of Geriatric Psychiatry and Neurology. 2018;**31**:319-328

[122] Vatter S, McDonald KR, Stanmore E, et al. A qualitative study of female

caregiving spouses' experiences of intimate relationships as cognition declines in Parkinson's disease. Age and Ageing. 2018;**47**:604-610

[123] Pozzebon M, Douglas J, Ames D. Spouses' experience of living with a partner diagnosed with a dementia: A synthesis of the qualitative research. International Psychogeriatrics. 2016;**28**:537-556

[124] Baxter LA, Braithwaite DO, Golish TD, Olson LN. Contradictions of interaction for wives of elderly husbands with adult dementia. Journal of Applied Communication Research. 2002;**30**:1-26

[125] Rollins D, Waterman D, Esmay D. Married widowhood. Activities, Adaptation, and Aging. 1985;7:67-71

[126] Davis LL, Gilliss CL, Deshefy-Longhi T, et al. The nature and scope of stressful spousal caregiving relationships. Journal of Family Nursing. 2011;**17**:224-240

[127] Boylstein C, Hayes J. Reconstructing marital closeness while caring for a spouse with Alzheimer's. Journal of Family Issues. 2012;**33**:584-612

[128] Massimo L, Evans LK, Benner P. Caring for loved ones with frontotemporal degeneration: The lived experiences of spouses. Geriatric Nursing. 2013;**34**:302-306

[129] Evans D, Lee E. Impact of dementia on marriage: A qualitative systematic review. Dementia. 2014;**13**:330-349

[130] Clark S, Prescott T, Murphy G. The lived experiences of dementia in married couple relationships. Dementia. 2017. https://doi.org/10.1177/1471301217722034

[131] Kaplan L. A couplehood typology for spouses of institutionalized persons with Alzheimer's disease: Perceptions of "We"–"I". Family Relations. 2001;**50**:87-98

[132] Sanders S, Power J. Roles, responsibilities and relationships among older husbands caring for wives with progressive dementia and other chronic conditions. Health and Social Work. 2009;**34**:41-51

[133] Shin H, Youn J, Kim JS, et al. Caregiver burden in Parkinson disease with dementia compared to Alzheimer disease in Korea. Journal of Geriatric Psychiatry and Neurology. 2012;**25**:222-226

[134] Svendsboe E, Terum T, Testad I, et al. Caregiver burden in family carers of people with dementia with Lewy bodies and Alzheimer's disease. International Journal of Geriatric Psychiatry. 2016;**31**:1075-1083

[135] Bjoerke-Bertheussen J, Ehrt U, Rongve A, et al. Neuropsychiatric symptoms in mild dementia with Lewy bodies and Alzheimer's disease. Dementia and Geriatric Cognitive Disorders. 2012;**34**:1-6

[136] Ricci M, Guidoni SV, Sepe-Monti M, et al. Clinical findings, functional abilities and caregiver distress in the early stage of dementia with Lewy bodies (DLB) and Alzheimer's disease (AD). Archives of Gerontology and Geriatrics. 2009;**49**:e101-e104

[137] Liu S, Liu J, Wang XD, et al. Caregiver burden, sleep quality, depression, and anxiety in dementia caregivers: A comparison of frontotemporal lobar degeneration, dementia with Lewy bodies, and Alzheimer's disease. International Psychogeriatrics. 2018;**30**:1131-1138

[138] Lee DR, McKeith I, Mosimann U, et al. Examining carer stress in dementia: The role of subtype diagnosis and neuropsychiatric symptoms.

International Journal of Geriatric Psychiatry. 2013;**28**:135-141

[139] Vatter S, Stanmore E, Clare L, et al. Care burden and mental ill health in spouses of people with Parkinson disease dementia and Lewy body dementia. Journal of Geriatric Psychiatry and Neurology. 2019. (in press)

[140] Zigmond AS, Snaith RP. The hospital anxiety and depression scale. Acta Psychiatrica Scandinavica. 1983;**67**:361-370

[141] Greene JG, Smith R, Gardiner M, Timbury GC. Measuring behavioural disturbance of elderly demented patients in the community and its effects on relatives: A factor analytic study. Age and Ageing. 1982;**11**:121-126

[142] Burns DD. Ten Days to Self-Esteem. New York: Quill William Morrow; 1983

[143] EuroQoL Group. EuroQol—A new facility for the measurement of health-related quality of life. Health Policy. 1990;**16**:199-208

[144] Schofield HL, Murphy B, Herrman HE, et al. Family caregiving: Measurement of emotional well-being and various aspects of the caregiving role. Psychological Medicine. 1997;**27**:647-657

[145] Grün D, Pieri V, Vaillant M, Diederich NJ. Contributory factors to caregiver burden in Parkinson disease. Journal of the American Medical Directors Association. 2016;**17**:626-632

[146] Croog SH, Burleson JA, Sudilovsky A, Baume RM. Spouse caregivers of Alzheimer patients: Problem responses to caregiver burden. Aging and Mental Health. 2006;**10**:87-100

[147] Parkinson M, Carr SM, Rushmer R, Abley C. Investigating what works to support family carers of people with dementia: A rapid realist review. Journal of Public Health. 2017;**39**:e290-e301

[148] Wu YT, Clare L, Hindle JV, et al. Dementia subtype and living well: Results from the improving the experience of dementia and enhancing active life (IDEAL) study. BMC Medicine. 2018;**16**:140

[149] NHS Digital, Adult Social Care Statistics Team. Personal Social Services Survey of Adult Carers in England (SACE), 2016-17. 2017. Available from: https://digital.nhs.uk/data-and-information/publications/statistical/personal-social-services-survey-of-adult-carers/personal-social-services-survey-of-adult-carers-in-england-2016-17#summary [Accessed: February 15, 2019]

[150] Fletcher GJO, Simpson JA, Thomas G. The measurement of perceived relationship quality components: A confirmatory factor analytic approach. Personality and Social Psychology Bulletin. 2000;**26**:340-354

[151] Spanier GB. The measurement of marital quality. Journal of Sex and Marital Therapy. 1979;**5**:288-300

[152] Kelley HH, Thibaut JW. Interpersonal Relations: A Theory of Interdependence. New York: John Wiley & Sons; 1978

[153] Thibaut JW, Kelley HH. The Social Psychology of Groups. New York: John Wiley & Sons; 1959

[154] Rusbult CE, Buunk BP. Commitment processes in close relationships: An interdependence analysis. Journal of Social and Personal Relationships. 1993;**10**:175-204

[155] Rusbult CE, Martz JM, Agnew CR. The investment model scale: Measuring commitment level, satisfaction level, quality of alternatives,

and investment size. Personal Relationships. 1998;**5**:357-391

[156] Hodgson JH, Garcia K, Tyndall L. Parkinson's disease and the couple relationship: A qualitative analysis. Families, Systems and Health. 2004;**22**:101-118

[157] Buhmann C, Dogas S, Vettorazzi E, et al. The impact of Parkinson disease on patients' sexuality and relationship. Journal of Neural Transmission. 2017;**124**:983-996

[158] Archbold PG, Stewart BJ, Greenlick MR, Harvath T. Mutuality and preparedness as predictors of caregiver role strain. Research in Nursing and Health. 1990;**13**:375-384

[159] Karlstedt M, Fereshtehnejad SM, Aarsland D, Lökk J. Determinants of dyadic relationship and its psychosocial impact in patients with Parkinson's disease and their spouses. Parkinson's Disease. 2017;**4697052**:1-9

[160] Basco MR, Prager KJ, Pita JM, et al. Communication and intimacy in the marriages of depressed patients. Journal of Family Psychology. 1992;**6**:184-194

[161] Morris LW, Morris RG, Britton PG. The relationship between marital intimacy, perceived strain and depression in spouse caregivers of dementia sufferers. The British Journal of Medical Psychology. 1988;**61**:231-236

[162] Mavandadi S, Dobkin R, Mamikonyan E, et al. Benefit finding and relationship quality in Parkinson's disease: A pilot dyadic analysis of husbands and wives. Journal of Family Psychology. 2014;**28**:728-734

[163] Tanji H, Anderson KE, Gruber-Baldini AL, et al. Mutuality of the marital relationship in Parkinson's disease. Movement Disorders. 2008;**23**:1843-1849

[164] Wright LK. Affection and sexuality in the presence of Alzheimer's disease: A longitudinal study. Sexuality and Disability. 1998;**16**:167-178

[165] Davies HD, Sridhar SB, Newkirk LA, et al. Gender differences in sexual behaviors of AD patients and their relationship to spousal caregiver well-being. Aging and Mental Health. 2012;**16**:89-101

[166] Habermann B. Spousal perspective of Parkinson's disease in middle life. Journal of Advanced Nursing. 2000;**31**:1409-1415

[167] Carter RE, Carter CA. Marital adjustment and effects of illness in married pairs with one or both spouses chronically ill. The American Journal of Family Therapy. 1994;**22**:315-326

[168] Vatter S. The impact of Parkinson's-related dementia on life partner outcomes [thesis]. Manchester: University of Manchester; 2018

Chapter 5

State of Art of Telemonitoring in Patients with Diabetes Mellitus, with a Focus on Elderly Patients

Emmanuel Andrès, Laurent Meyer, Abrar-Ahmad Zulfiqar, Mohamed Hajjam, Samy Talha, Sylvie Ervé, Jawad Hajjam, Nathalie Jeandidier and Amir Hajjam El Hassani

Abstract

Since the beginning of the 1990s, several telemedicine projects and studies focused on type 1 and type 2 diabetes have been developed, including very few elderly diabetic patients. Several of these projects specifically concerned elderly subjects (n = 4). Mainly, these projects and studies show that telemonitoring diabetes results in improved blood glucose control—a significant reduction in HbA1c, improved patient ownership of the disease, greater patient adherence to therapeutic and hygiene-dietary measures, positive impact on comorbidities (hypertension, weight, dyslipidemia), improved quality of life for patients, and at least good patient receptivity and accountability. To date, the magnitude of its effects remains debatable, especially with the variation in patients' characteristics (e.g., background, ability for self-management, medical condition), sample selection, and approach for treatment of control groups. Over the last 5 years, numerous telemedicine projects based on connected objects and new information and communication technologies (ICT) (elements defining telemedicine 2.0) have emerged or are still under development.

Keywords: elderly patient, telemedicine, telemonitoring, diabetes, artificial intelligence, information and communication technology, Web, heart failure, chronic disease

1. Introduction

Intensive glucose control has been shown to delay or prevent the development of micro- and macrovascular complications related to diabetes, even in elderly diabetic patients. However, it is estimated that 43.2–55.6% of diabetic patients with type 2 diabetes do not meet the reference target for glycemic control (hemoglobin A1c [HbA1c] < 7.0%) [1]. Factors that may contribute to suboptimal blood glucose (BG) control include inadequate home BG monitoring, nonadherence or noncompliance with medications or lifestyle changes (nutrition and sport), suboptimal patient education about the disease, and limited access to health professionals [1–3]. In the absence of timely and accurate data on home BG values, healthcare professionals may be reluctant, rightly so, to aggressively intensify oral hypoglycemic agents or insulin treatments for fear of hypoglycemia [4].

This is particularly true in the elderly, where hypoglycemia can have dramatic consequences, such as myocardial infarction (MI), falls, etc. These patients have a high mortality rate, with 20% of deaths occurring within 5 years after the first cardiovascular event. In this context, patients are often hospitalized, with prolonged and iterative hospitalization [2].

In practice, the main causes of diabetes required medical intervention are related to the following: nontherapeutic adherence and compliance, poor nutrition, and poor adherence to prescribed lifestyle changes and therapy, the decompensation of diabetic comorbidities and macrovascular complication, and community-based infections [2]. In this context, telemedicine may be an effective approach in solving problems of education, compliance, and monitoring and provider access [2, 5]. BG control could be safely improved by basing drug changes on home BG readings and transmitting them in near real time to providers, particularly in elderlies. In this setting, telemedicine may also be an effective solution to monitor the complications of the diabetes, especially macrovascular complications (e.g., MI, heart failure [HF], etc.) and comorbidities (e.g., arterial hypertension).

In this article, we review the literature in the field of telemonitoring (remote monitoring) of diabetic patients, with a focus on elderly diabetic patients.

2. First-generation telemedicine projects and studies in the field of diabetes

Since the early 1990s to the end of 2010, numerous telemedicine projects and studies have been developed in the field of diabetes [6–27]. Practically all of them have investigated *telemonitoring* or *telephone follow-up* (defined terms in **Table 1**), especially to monitor BG levels. For the majority of them, they were conducted on specific population of poor controlled type 1 and type 2 diabetic patients, including very few elderly diabetic patients. Several of these projects include specifically elderly diabetic patients (< 80 years old) (n = 1) [21, 27]. Mainly these projects have been developed in children and young people (n = 3), young or mild-age patients with intensified therapy (n = 2), young or mild-age patients under insulin pump therapy (n = 1), and patients with complicated or complex diabetes, including several elderly patients (n = 2) [6–27].

To our knowledge, to date, no project has been published on *tele-consultation* and *teleexpertise* (defined terms in **Table 1**) in the area of diabetes domain, as defined under European or French legislation [28]. Several of such projects have been developed, but no formal scientific conclusions are currently available about the usefulness of these telemedicine technologies [29].

It is worth bearing in mind that these projects and studies [6–27], particularly the earlier ones, more closely resembled as a telephone follow-up with care providers (such as a nurse) traveling to the diabetic patient's home rather than telemedicine use as we think of it nowadays with nonintrusive, automated, smart telemonitoring employing remote sensors via modern communication technology (e.g., smartphone) or even artificial intelligence (AI) (**Table 1**) [29]. Thus, they characterize in our opinion *first-generation* telemedicine projects and studies.

Using *PubMed* database and *Google Scholar*, we have identified more than 20 reports of first-generation telemonitoring studies in the field of diabetes, including type 1 and type 2 diabetic patients, involving the upload and direct transmission of BG data by diabetic patients to providers via cellular telephone, telephone landline, or a Web-based program [6–27]. The results of these studies were mixed, perhaps because many studies did not target diabetic patients with poor baseline BG control or the interval between glucose transmission and follow-up was delayed or unspecified or mainly with no therapeutic intervention (therapeutic inertia). None of these

-**Telemedicine**: provision of remote patient care and consultation using telecommunication technologies.
-**Telemonitoring**: this telemedicine practice allows a healthcare professional to remotely interpret the data necessary for the patient's medical follow-up in order to make decisions about his / her care. Remote data collection from a patient through a connected device or questionnaires to monitor his/her vital parameters and symptoms at home on a daily basis.
-**Teleexpertise**: this practice of telemedicine consists, for a medical professional, to seek the opinion of one or more medical professional experts regarding elements of the patient's medical file. Remote seeking by a health professional of a second medical opinion via sending of images (scanner, X-ray, eye fundus, etc.) and sometimes exchange by Internet-based videoconference.
-**Teleconsultation**: this telemedicine practice allows a medical professional to hold a consultation with a patient remotely. In the context of a teleconsultation, the patient can have at his/her side a health professional assisting the remote professional as well as a psychologist. Second opinion consultation by specialist.
-**Telemedicine 2.0**: over the last decade, the Internet has become increasingly popular and is now an important part of our daily life. The use of "Web 2.0" technologies in health/medicine care or in telemedicine is referred to as "Health 2.0" or "Medicine 2.0," and "telemedicine 2.0."
-**Artificial intelligence**: this concept makes it possible for machines to learn from experience, adjust to new inputs and perform human-like tasks. These processes include learning (the acquisition of information and rules for using the information), reasoning (using the rules to reach approximate or definite conclusions) and self-correction. Particular applications of AI include expert systems, speech recognition, and machine vision.

Table 1.
Glossary of terms and definitions in the field of telemedicine [29].

reports evaluated the intensity of intervention required to sustain achieved reductions in HbA1c after the implementation of home telemonitoring.

As with CHF, the results of these first-generation telemedicine projects differed from study to study, with fairly inconclusive results as to their potential clinical benefits in terms of balancing diabetes and the associated metabolic problems, re-hospitalization, and decreased morbidity or mortality, particularly regarding the statistical significance of the results [29, 30]. As a consequence, experts have shared now widely divergent opinions on the actual utility of telemedicine in diabetic patient management [29, 30].

To our knowledge, it should be emphasized that the first-generation studies and trials on telemedicine in diabetic patients were at times conducted with [29]:

- Inappropriate methodologies, involving unsuitable patient groups (such as well-balanced diabetic patients, diabetic patients without any complication) of small-sized patient samples and with very short follow-up periods (between 3 months and 1 year)

- Not well-structured follow-up organization, with nonspecialized staff to alarms, or without any association of patients' general practitioners, specialists of diabetes management, or endocrinologists nor any optimized management process or algorithm

- Several alarms arising too late, without therapeutic response (no specified therapeutic protocol available)

- No associated educational programs

- The absence of a human interface or contact between the telemedicine solution and the patients

Moreover, most of these studies were only based on glycemic control, without including other warning or monitoring parameters related to comorbidities or diabetic complication (e.g., tensiometer, heart rate, balance), with an underutilization

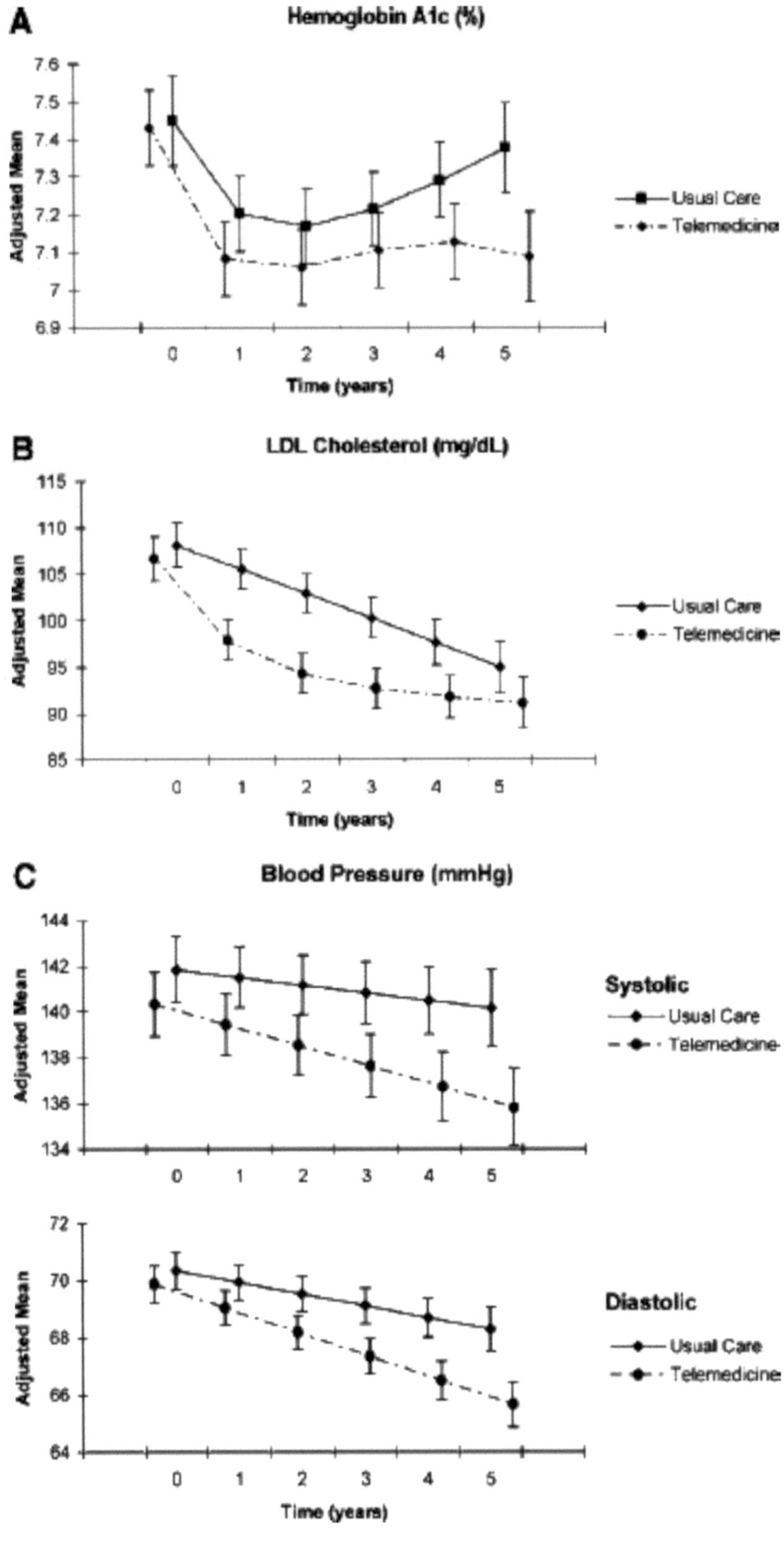

Figure 1.
Results of IDEAtel trial (n = 1665 diabetic elderly patients) (adapted from [21, 27]).

of the deployed device [29, 30]. Thus in our opinion, these facts explain that the demonstration of any benefits with these first-generation studies was "illusory," in particular in terms of statistical significance.

Besides these medical considerations, it is worth noting that an economical aspect must be investigated and consolidated in future telemedicine projects to promote the development of telemedicine in diabetes and legitimize it, especially in regard of the budgetary constraints affecting insurance and mutual health insurance companies. Things are less advanced than in the field of chronic heart failure telemonitoring [29]. To our knowledge, only Biermann's study is dedicated to this theme of economical aspect [11].

To date, none of the learned societies (e.g., *American Diabetes Association* [ADA], *European Society of Diabetes* [ESD]) involved in the topic of diabetes has, to our knowledge, made any formal recommendation as to whether or not telemedicine is of benefit to type 1 or type 2 diabetic patients. This is not the case in the setting of CHF, where factual data and medico-economic studies are more numerous, better documented, and consolidated (more mature field) [29]. In fact, the 2016 *European Society of Cardiology* (ESC) guidelines for the diagnosis and treatment of acute and chronic heart failure have recommended telemonitoring of heart failure patients with a recommendation grade of IIb and level of evidence B [31].

In the setting of diabetic patients, Shea et al. have conducted the first telemedicine study specifically dedicated to "elderly" diabetic patients (aged 55 years or greater) [21, 27]. It is a randomized, controlled trial comparing telemedicine case management to usual care, with blinding of those obtaining outcome data, in 1665 Medicare recipients with diabetes. In the intervention group (n = 844), mean HbA1c improved over 1 year from 7.35 to 6.97% and from 8.35 to 7.42% in the subgroup with baseline HbA1c $\geq$ 7% (n = 353) [21]. In the usual care group (n = 821), mean HbA1c improved over 1 year from 7.42 to 7.17%. Adjusted net reductions (1 year minus baseline mean values in each group, compared between groups) favoring the intervention were as follows (all principal criteria): HbA1c, 0.18% ($p = 0.006$); systolic and diastolic blood pressure, 3.4 ($p = 0.001$) and 1.9 mmHg ($p < 0.001$); and LDL cholesterol, 9.5 mg/dL ($p < 0.001$) (**Figure 1**). In the subgroup with baseline HbA1c $\geq$ 7%, net adjusted reduction in HbA1c favoring the intervention group was 0.32% ($p = 0.002$). Mean LDL cholesterol level in the intervention group at 1 year was 95.7 mg/dL. Mortality was not different between the groups, although power was limited. There were 176 deaths in the intervention group and 169 in the usual care group (hazard ratio 1.01 [0.82, 1.24]).

3. Second-generation telemedicine projects and studies in the field of diabetes

Over the last 10 years, *second-generation* telemedicine projects and studies have been developed in the setting of diabetes management, especially in the setting of telemonitoring [32–38], as defined in **Table 1**. These projects and studies have main objectives to evaluate the use of technology to implement medical and cost-effective healthcare management on a large scale for diabetes management. These projects include very few elderly patients. One project, the DiaTel study, was dedicated to elderly diabetic patients (<80 years old) [32]. Compared to the aforementioned project, most of the second-generation projects related to diabetes telemonitoring (for type 1 diabetic patients, n = 1; for type 2, n = 5) incorporate the following [32–38]:

- Self-administered medical questionnaires or forms on symptoms and signs of diabetes decompensation and BG levels

- Tools for medical education, particularly disease self-appropriation, food hygiene, and physical activity
- Tools for patient motivation
- Tools for therapeutic and hygiene observance
- Tool to remote comorbidities (e.g., arterial hypertension, obesity, dyslipidemia)
- Tools for interaction between the patient and healthcare professionals like telephone support centers, tablets, and Websites

3.1 The DiaTel study

The DiaTel study compared the short-term efficacy of home telemonitoring coupled with active medication management by a nurse practitioner with a monthly care coordination telephone call on glycemic control in veterans with type 2 diabetes [32]. The included patients were taking oral hypoglycemic agents and/or insulin for ≥1 year and had HbA1c ≥ 7.5%). Approximately one-third of the participants in both groups were aged 65 years. At enrollment, the patients were randomly assigned to either active care management (AMC) with home telemonitoring (HT) (ACM + HT group, n = 73) or a monthly care coordination telephone call (CC group, n = 77) [32]. Both groups received monthly calls for DM education and self-management review. ACM + HT group participants transmitted BG, blood pressure (BP), and weight to a nurse practitioner; the nurse practitioner adjusted medications for glucose, BP, and lipid control based on established ADA targets. Baseline characteristics of the patients in the DiaTel study were similar in both groups, with mean HbA1c of 9.4% in the CC group vs. 9.6% in ACM + HT group [32, 33]. Compared with the CC group, the ACM + HT group demonstrated significantly larger decreases in HbA1c (principal criterion) at 3 months (1.7 vs. 0.7%) and 6 months (1.7 vs. 0.8%; $p < 0.001$ for each), with most improvement occurring by 3 months (**Figure 2**).

3.2 The Utah Remote Monitoring Project

The Utah Remote Monitoring Project was a nonrandomized prospective observational pre- and post-intervention study [34]. The included patients were patients with uncontrolled type 2 diabetes and/or arterial hypertension. They have been enrolled from four rural and two urban primary care clinics and one urban stroke center participated in a telemonitoring program (n = 109). The primary clinical outcome measures were changes in HbA1c and BP. Other outcomes included fasting lipids, weight, patient engagement, diabetes knowledge, arterial hypertension knowledge, medication adherence, and patient perceptions of the usefulness of the telemonitoring program. The patients were randomized in two groups on telemonitoring delivery methods [34]. The first was a remote monitoring device for BP and heart rate. Patients used their own glucose meters to measure BG and were provided with an electronic digital scale to measure their weight. The device was programmed to sound an alarm at a pre-specified patient-referred time to prompt the patient to initiate a telemonitoring session. Patients were asked to enter data several times during the week. The device was programmed to ask how patients were feeling that day and whether they had taken their medications and then receive a prompt to take the measures. After, the patient received a series of education messages, focused on teaching patients about their diseases (diabetes, arterial

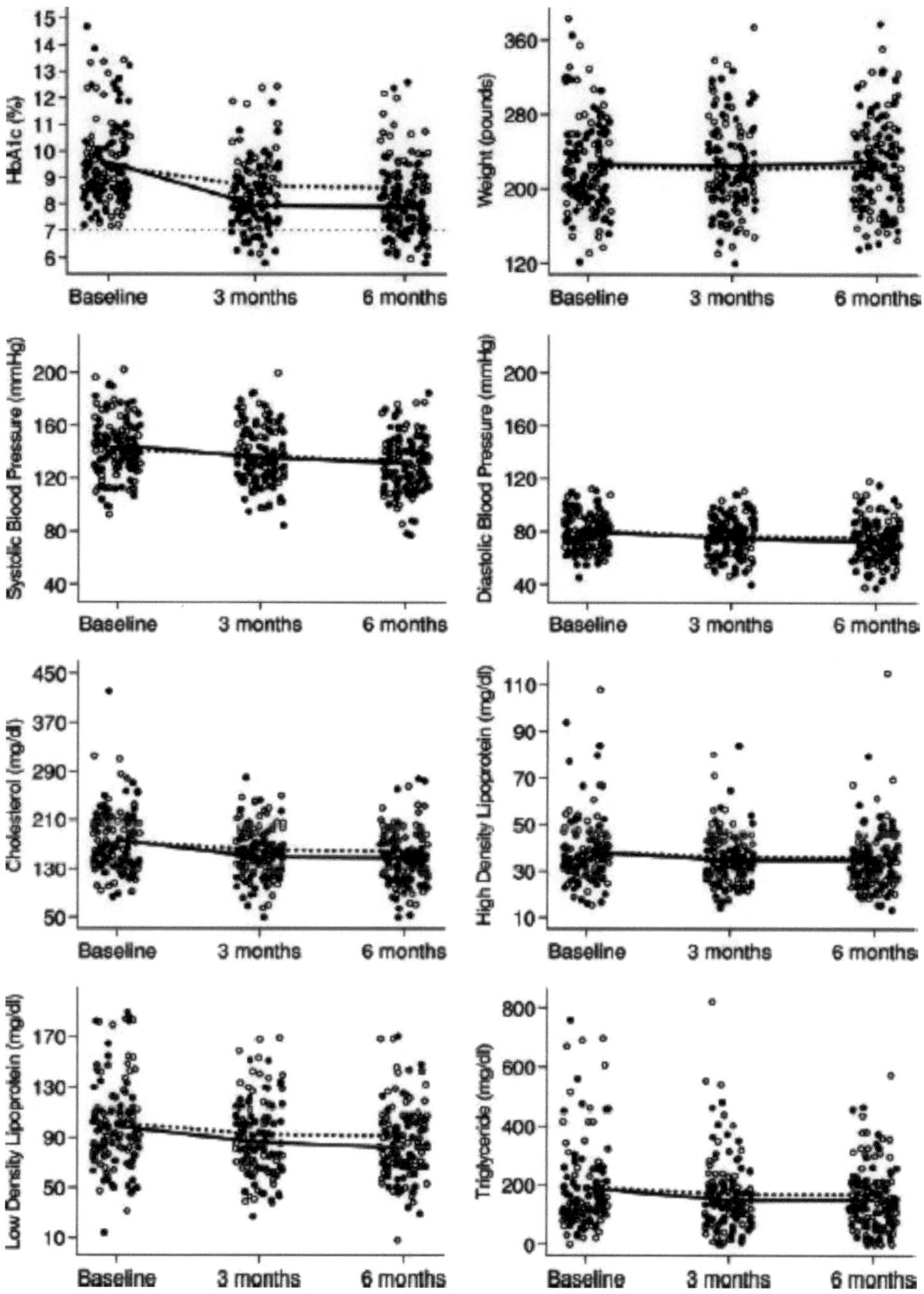

Figure 2.
Results of DiaTel study (n = 150 diabetic elderly patients) (adapted from [32]).

hypertension) and associated comorbidities. The second telemonitoring delivery method is the use of an interactive voice response (IVR) system. Patients were provided with a BP monitor and electronic digital scales, but they used their own BG meter. The patients have to use the same process described above, but received a call from the telemonitoring IVR service at a pre-specified. Medical providers were contacted either via a note in the electronic medical record (or immediately if there was a concern, in person or by telephone) if there was an out-of-range value (decided by individual providers or clinics as a value that was high or low). In this study, the mean HbA1c (principal criterion) decreased: 9.73% at baseline vs.

7.81% at the end of the program ($p < 0.0001$) [34]. Systolic BP (principal criterion) also declined significantly: 130.7 mmHg at baseline vs. 122.9 mmHg at the end ($p = 0.0001$). Low-density lipoprotein content decreased significantly: 103.9 mg/dL at baseline vs. 93.7 mg/dL at the end ($p = 0.0263$). Knowledge of diabetes and arterial hypertension increased significantly ($p < 0.001$ for both). Patient engagement and medication adherence also improved, but not significantly. Per questionnaires at study end, patients felt the telemonitoring program was useful.

3.3 Randomized trial on home telemonitoring for the management of metabolic and cardiovascular risk in patients with type 2 diabetes

This study evaluated whether a home telehealth (HT) system can improve metabolic control and overall cardiovascular risk in individuals with type 2 diabetes, compared with usual practice [35]. This study was a randomized, parallel-group, open-label, multicenter study conducted in general practice (29 general practitioners) including 302 patients, with a follow-up of 12 months. The HT system (for the telemedicine group of diabetic patients, n = 153) offers to the patient the possibility to monitor body weight, BG values, and BP values, associated with remote educational support and feedback to the general practitioner [35]. The use of the HT system was associated with a statistically significant reduction in HbA1c levels (principal criterion) compared with the control group: estimated mean difference of 0.33 ± 0.1 ($p = 0.001$) [35]. No difference was documented for body weight, BP, and lipid profile (all principal criteria). The proportion of patients reaching the target of HbA1c (HbA1c < 7.0%) was higher in the HT group than in the control group after 6 months, 33.0 vs. 18.7% ($p = 0.009$), and 12 months, 28.1 vs. 18.5% ($p = 0.07$). As for quality of life (evaluated with the 36-item short-form health survey), significant differences in favor of the HT group were detected as for physical functioning ($p = 0.01$) and mental health ($p = 0.005$). On an economic level, a lower number of specialist visits was reported in the telemedicine group: incidence rate ratio of 0.72 (95% confidence interval, 0.51–1.01; $p = 0.06$).

3.4 Study assessed the utility and cost-effectiveness of an automated Diabetes Remote Monitoring and Management System (DRMS)

This study assessed the utility and cost-effectiveness of an automated Diabetes Remote Monitoring and Management System (DRMS) in glycemic control versus usual care [36]. In this randomized, controlled study, patients with uncontrolled diabetes on insulin were randomized to use the DRMS or usual care. Participants in both groups were followed up for 6 months and had three clinic visits during the study period (at 0, 3, and 6 months [35]). The DRMS used text messages or phone calls to remind patients to test their BG and to report results via an automated system, with no human interaction unless a patient had severely high or low BG. The DRMS made adjustments to insulin dose(s) based on validated algorithms. Participants reported medication adherence through the Morisky Medication Adherence Scale-8, and diabetes-specific quality of life through the diabetes daily quality-of-life questionnaire. A cost-effectiveness analysis was conducted based on the estimated overall costs of DRMS and usual care. A total of 98 diabetic patients (60% of female) treated with insulin therapy were enrolled [36]. The mean age of the patients was 59 years. At the end, 87 patients (89%) have completed the follow-up. HbA1c was similar between the DRMS and control groups at 3 months, 7.60 vs. 8.10%, and at 6 months, 8.10 vs. 7.90% (p = ns) (principal criterion) [42]. Changes from baseline to 6 months were not statistically significant for self-reported medication adherence and diabetes-specific quality of life, except for the Daily Quality of Life-Social/Vocational Concerns subscale score ($p = 0.04$).

3.5 The Telescot Diabetes Pragmatic Multicenter Randomized Controlled Trial

The Telescot Diabetes is a randomized, parallel, investigator-blind controlled trial with centralized randomization in family practices in four regions of the United Kingdom [37]. This study included 321 patients with relatively well-controlled type 2 diabetes, with an HbA1c > 7.46%. In Telescot Diabetes, 160 people were randomized to the intervention group and 161 to the usual care group [37]. The supported telemonitoring intervention involved self-measurement and transmission to a secure Website of twice-weekly morning and evening glucose for review by family practice clinicians who were not blinded to allocation group. The control group received usual care, with at least annual review and more frequent reviews for people with poor glycemic or BP control. HbA1c assessed at ninth month was the primary outcome. The mean (SD) HbA1c at follow-up was 7.92% in the intervention group vs. 8.36% in the usual care group [37]. For primary analysis, adjusted mean HbA1c was 0.51% lower (95% CI 0.22% to 0.81%, (principal criterion) (p = 0.0007)). For secondary analyses, adjusted mean ambulatory systolic BP was 3.06 mmHg lower (95% CI 0.56–5.56 mmHg, p = 0.017) and mean ambulatory diastolic BP was 2.17 mmHg lower (95% CI 0.62–3.72, p = 0.006) among people in the intervention group when compared with usual care after adjustment. No significant differences were identified between groups in weight, treatment pattern, adherence to medication, or quality of life in secondary analyses. During the study, the number of telephone calls was greater between nurses and patients in the intervention compared with control group: rate ratio of 7.50 (95% CI 4.45–12.65, p < 0.0001), but no other significant differences between groups in the use of health services were identified between groups.

3.6 Educ@dom

Educ@dom is a multicenter, randomized, controlled, prospective study [38]. The primary objective of this study is to compare the efficacy of telemonitoring to standard monitoring in terms of changes in HbA1c after a 1-year follow-up period. The secondary objectives are clinical (changes in knowledge, physical activity, weight, etc.) and medical-economic. The Educ@dom study included 282 patients, 141 patients in each arm [38]. For patients in the intervention group, the device will be given to them for 1 year and then withdrawn during the second year of follow-up. The anticipated benefits of this research are an improvement in BG management in patients with type 2 diabetes by improving their lifestyle while rationalizing recourse to consultations in order to reduce the incidence of complications and cost in the long term. The results of this study are expected in 2019–2020.

4. New-generation projects and studies in diabetes

Over the last 5 years, new-generation telemedicine projects and studies have emerged in the setting of chronic diseases setting, especially in the setting of chronic heart failure, chronic obstructive pulmonary diseases, and type 1 and type 2 diabetes [29, 39–42]. They support transmission and remote interpretation of patients' data for follow-up and preventive interventions. These projects and studies have for main objectives to evaluate the use of technology to implement medical and cost-effective healthcare management on a large scale for diabetes management. Using *PubMed* database and *Google Scholar*, we have identified three of such projects and studies in the field of diabetes management: Telemonitoring and Health Counseling for Self-Management Support from Lindberg et al.,

TELESAGE, and DIABETe [39–42]. All these projects include elderly diabetic patients. Of note for the first time, one the telemedicine projects developed for chronic diseases management, the TIM-HF2 study [43], has recently demonstrated the usefulness of telemedicine in chronic heart failure, with statistical significance, in a prospective randomized study (the *gold standard* of evidence-based medicine [EBM]).

Between August 13, 2013, and May 12, 2017, 1571 patients (mean age of 70 years) were included in the TIM-HF2 study and randomly assigned to remote patient management (n = 796) or standard care (n = 775) [43]. At baseline, all patients exhibited a left ventricular ejection fraction of <45% and NYHA II or III while receiving treatment with diuretics. In TIM-HF2 study, the percentage of days lost due to unplanned cardiovascular hospital admissions and all-cause death was 4.88% (95% CI 4.55–5.23) in the remote patient management group vs. 6.64% (6.19–7.13) in the standard care group (ratio 0.80, 95% CI: 0.65–1) (p = 0.0460). The all-cause death rate was 7.86 (95% CI: 6.14–10.10) per 100 person-years of follow-up in the remote patient management group vs. 11.34 (95% CI: 9.21–13.95) per 100 person-years of follow-up in the standard care group (hazard ratio [HR] 0.70, 95% CI: 0.5–0.96) (p = 0.0280) (**Figure 3**). Cardiovascular mortality did not significantly differ between both groups (HR 0.671, 95% CI: 0.45–1.01; p = 0.056).

The TIM-HF2 study utilized a noninvasive, multiparameter telemonitoring system installed in the patient's home, comprising a three-channel ECG, BP-monitoring device, and weighing scales, by means of which the information was transferred remotely [43]. Patients received a mobile phone in order to contact the telemedical center in case of emergency. Patients were likewise followed via monthly phone interviews. For this TIM-HF2 care strategy, the key component was a well-structured telemedical center with physicians and HF nurses (*center of coordination*), available 24 hours a day and every day a week, able to act promptly according to the individual patient risk profile. The actions taken by the telemedical center staff included changes in medication and admission to hospital, as needed, in addition to educational activities.

In this setting, we believe that, thanks to technological innovations in connected health-monitoring devices, the telemonitoring of type 2 diabetic patients using

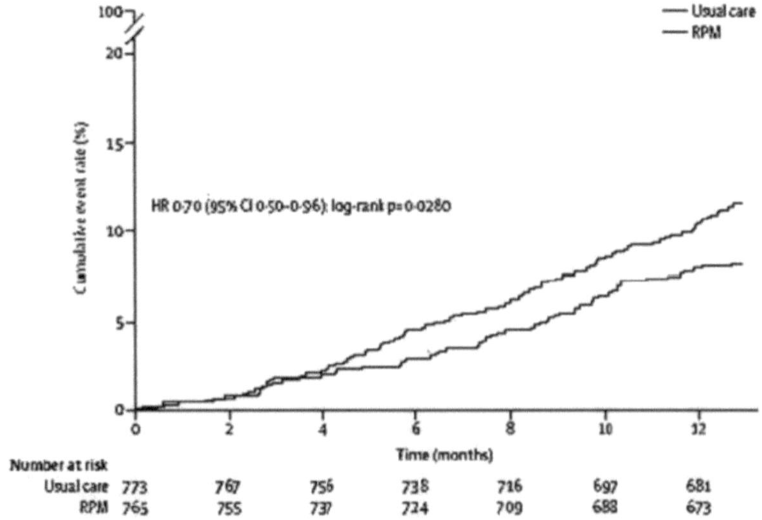

Figure 3.
TIM-HF2 trial. Rate of cumulative events in patients randomly assigned to remote patient management (n = 796) or usual care (n = 775) (adapted from [43]).

therapeutic educational tools is likely to help them adapt to their treatment and lifestyle habits and therefore improve BG management [29].

These new-generation telemedicine projects in diabetes (Telemonitoring and Health Counseling for Self-Management Support from Lindberg et al., TELESAGE, DIABETe) [39–42] are often known as *telemedicine 2.0* projects, given that they all utilize new information and communication technologies (ICT) and the Web (tools for the *e-Health 2.0*) (as defined in **Table 1**) [44].

Most projects and studies rely on the standard connected tools for monitoring type 1 and type 2 diabetes, such as glucose meters, BP, heart rate monitors, weighing scales, and pulse oximeters, which relay the collected information via Bluetooth, 3G, or 4G [29, 39–42]. Several projects also include continuous glycemic monitoring solution and often a video-call [29, 30]. Several of these telemedicine projects use machine learning, also called artificial intelligence (AI), in order to be able to:

- Adjust the BG level to the patient's activity (software Diabeo™ [see below]) [40, 41].

- Predict patient risks of diabetes decompensation [42, 45]. In this later situation, the cloud-based software aggregates, cleans, and analyzes patient data to allow for identifying patterns that may indicate potential risks and provide predictive insights on healthcare outcomes, as the software MyPredi™ (see below) [29, 42].

In the setting of chronic diseases, as in chronic heart disease or in diabetes, several informatics solutions or tools have been developed and used, such as artificial neural network (ANN) algorithms, data mining software, and ontology [45, 46]. In this context of AI, three clinical datasets are of particular interest: (1) patients' phenotype; (2) patients' electronic medical records containing physicians' notes, laboratory test results, as well as other information on diseases, treatments, and epidemiology that may be of interest for association studies and predictive modeling on prognosis and drug responses; and (3) literature knowledge including rules on diabetes management [46].

Besides these tools, it must be emphasized that diabetes telemonitoring may use, as for CHF telemonitoring, implantable invasive devices that send either sporadically or continuously data to the receiving physician (automatic telemonitoring) (*outside the scope of this paper*) [30]. In management of diabetes, implantable telemonitoring devices for multiparameters including mainly BG-insulin levels monitoring have recently proven to be an effective approach.

4.1 Telemonitoring and Health Counseling for Self-Management Support of Patients with Type 2 Diabetes

The objective of this study (Telemonitoring and Health Counseling for Self-Management Support) was to investigate whether the introduction of a health technology-supported self-management program involving telemonitoring and health counseling had beneficial effects on HbA1c, other clinical variables (weight, body mass index, BP, blood lipid profile), and health-related quality of life (HRQoL), as measured using the short-form health survey (SF-36) version 2 in patients with type 2 diabetes [39]. This was a pragmatic randomized controlled trial of patients with type 2 diabetes. Both the control (n = 79) and intervention groups (n = 87) received usual care [39]. The intervention group also participated in additional health promotion activities with the use of the Prescribed Healthcare Web application for self-monitoring of BG and BP. About every second month or when needed, the general practitioner or the DM nurse reviewed the results and the healthcare activity plan. Analyses of the data showed that there were no significant differences between the groups in the primary outcome HbA1c level ($p = 0.33$) and in the secondary outcome HRQoL as measured using SF-36 [39]. A total of 80% of the patients in the intervention group at the baseline and 98% of the responders after 19-month intervention were familiar with using a personal computer ($p = 0.001$). After 19 months, no responders reported significantly poorer mental health in social functioning and role emotional subscales on the SF-36 ($p = 0.03$ and $p = 0.01$, respectively).

4.2 TELESAGE study

TELESAGE (*Suivi A Grande Echelle d'une population de diabétiques de type 1 et de type 2 sous schéma insulinique basal bolus par la TELEmédecine* [large-scale follow-up of a population of type 1 and type 2 diabetics under basal insulin regimen bolus by telemedicine]) is a 6-month open-label parallel-group, multicenter study, including adult patients (n = 180) with type 1 diabetes (>1 year), on a basal-bolus insulin regimen (> 6 months), with HbA1c ≥ 8%, conducted in approximately 100 centers in France [40, 41]. These type 1 diabetic patients were randomized to usual quarterly follow-up (G1), home use of a smartphone recommending insulin doses (Diabeo™ software) with quarterly visits (G2), or the use of the smartphone with short teleconsultations every 2 weeks but no visit until point end (G3) [40, 41]. The primary objective of TELESAGE will be to investigate the effect of the Diabeo™ telemedicine system versus usual follow-up, with respect to improvements in the HbA1c levels (principal criterion) of diabetic patients with poorly controlled basal-bolus insulin levels (n = 696). The study will compare a control group (group 1 [G1], usual follow-up) with two Diabeo™ telemedicine systems: (1) physician-assisted telemedicine (group 2 [G2]) and (2) nurse-assisted telemonitoring and teleconsultations by a diabetologist's task delegation (group 3 [G3]). At 6 months, the mean HbA1c level is as follows: 8.41 ± 1.04% in G3 vs. 8.63 ± 1.07% in G2 vs. 9.10 ± 1.16% in G1 ($p = 0.0019$ for G1–G3 comparison) (**Figure 4**) [40, 41]. The Diabeo™ system gave a 0.91% (0.60–1.21) improvement in HbA1c over controls and a 0.67% (0.35–0.99) reduction when used without teleconsultation. There was no difference in the frequency of hypoglycemic episodes or in medical time spent for hospital or telephone consultations. However, patients in G1 and G2 spent nearly 5 h more than G3 patients attending hospital visits.

4.3 DIABETe project

The DIABETe project is scheduled to experiment a telemonitoring solution for at-home monitoring of type 1 and type 2 diabetic patients [29, 42]. The DIABETe telemonitoring project, conducted in Strasbourg (France), falls under the "telemedicine 2.0" category (as described above) [29, 44]. It has been developed and designed to optimize home monitoring of diabetic patients by detecting, via a telemonitoring 2.0 platform, situations with a risk of decompensation of diabetes and its complications (e.g., MI or CHF), the latter ultimately leading to hospitalization [29, 42]. The AI of the DIABETe platform (MyPredi™) automatically generates indicators of *health status* deterioration, i.e., *warning alerts* for any chronic disease worsening, particularly diabetes, its macrovascular complications, and cardiovascular comorbidities (e.g., arterial hypertension, chronic heart failure). For the patient, these situations may lead to hospitalization if not treated appropriately. To our knowledge, this is one of the first projects that use AI in addition to ICT. The platform comprises connected nonintrusive medical sensors (**Figure 5**), a touchscreen tablet connected by Wi-Fi, and a router or 3G/4G, rendering it possible to interact with the patient and provide education on treatment, diet, and lifestyle [29, 42].

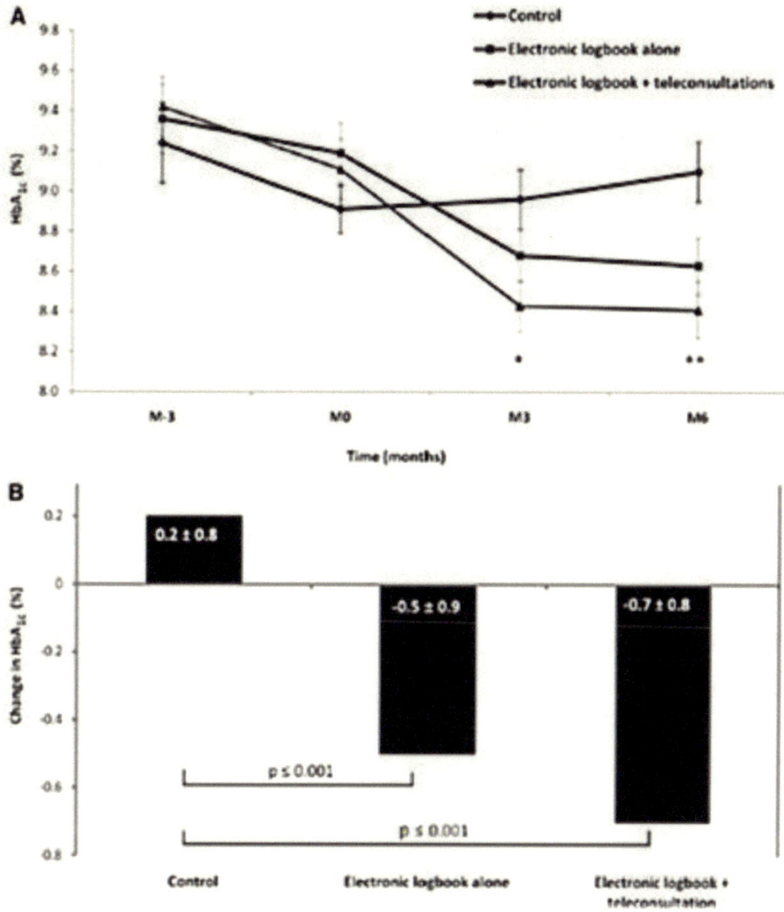

Figure 4.
Efficacy of the software Diabeo™ (adapted from [40]).

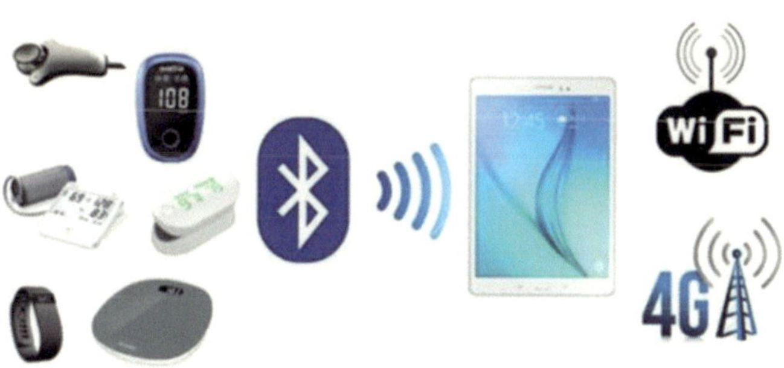

Figure 5.
DIABETe's connected nonintrusive medical sensors.

The system (**Figure 6**) involves a server that hosts the patient's data and a secure Internet portal to which the patient and hospital- and nonhospital-based healthcare professionals can connect (**Figure 7**) [29, 42].

DIABETe is based on a smart system comprising an inference engine and a medical ontology for personalized synchronous or asynchronous analysis of data specific to each patient and, if necessary, the sending of an AI-generated alert (MyPredi™) [29, 42].

DIABETe is run by a group bringing together the Strasbourg University Hospital (*Hôpitaux Universitaires de Strasbourg*), East Regional Health Agency (*Agence*

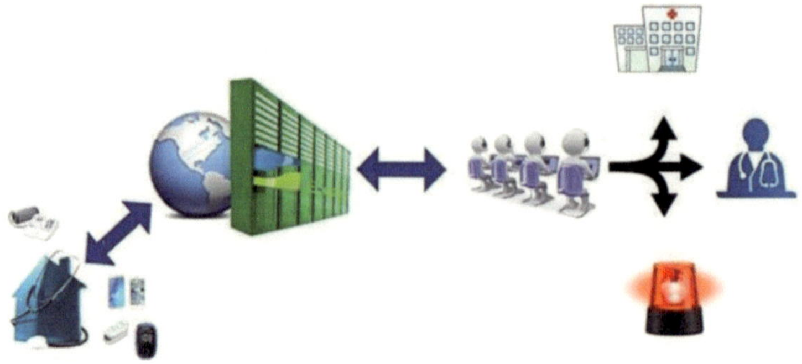

Figure 6.
DIABETe's platform.

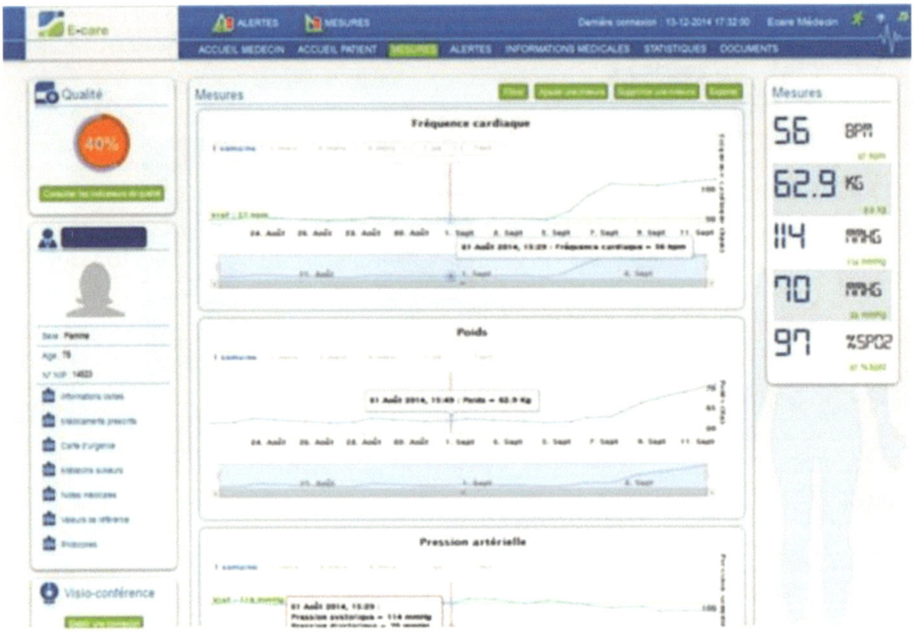

Figure 7.
DIABETe's Internet portal.

Régionale de Santé du Grand Est), Bas-Rhin branch of France's National Health Insurance (*Caisse Primaire d'Assurance du Bas-Rhin*), and *Predimed Technology* start-up [29, 42]. This project is likely allowing an in-depth study to be carried out designed to improve diagnosis by machine learning and detect abnormalities in diabetic patients at an early time point.

The telemonitoring platform used in DIABETe was first validated in a monocentric study conducted in the Strasbourg University Hospital, carried out as part of the E-Care project, primarily focused on the problem of CHF [47, 48]. Between February 2014 and April 2015, 175 elderly patients (mean age of 72 years) were included into the E-care project; 30% of these patients suffered from type 2 diabetes. During this period, the telemonitoring platform was used on a daily basis by patients and healthcare professionals, according to a defined protocol of use specific to each patient. During the study, 1500 measurements were taken, generating 700 alerts in 68 patients. One hundred seven subjects (61.1%) had no alerts upon follow-up. Analysis of the warning alerts in the 68 other patients showed that MyPredi™

detected any worsening of the "patient's health," with a sensitivity, specificity, as well as positive and negative predictive values of 100, 30, 89, and 100%, respectively. In this experimentation, both the healthcare professionals and patients, even the frailest, used the E-care system without difficulty until the end of the study.

The patients included in the DIABETe project were real-life type 1 and type 2 diabetic patients (n = 100) with (i) a "very high cardiovascular risk," when presenting a personal history of myocardial infarction or stroke, limb amputation, or cardiomyopathy and (ii) an "intensive" insulin therapy, with at least three injections per day or pump administration while offering them a personalized follow-up and education about their illness and its management [29, 42]. To date, several patients have been included. The results of this project are expected in late 2019–early 2020.

The DIABETe project is based on an intelligent platform that likely assists healthcare professionals by automatically processing the information obtained from nonintrusive medical sensors (BG meter, BP monitor, actimeter, connected scale, etc.) as well as the subjective information provided by the patient himself (questionnaires) and his/her behavior (compliance), enabling it to detect and report, at an early time, these situations at risk of hospitalization [29, 42]. Patient- and situation-adapted therapeutic education tools will be made available to the individual, and communication with the subject will likely occur via a touch pad. Alerts indicating a deterioration of the patient's condition will be generated by AI (new software version of MyPredi™ adapted for the management of diabetes) and transmitted to the health professionals in charge of the patient. The healthcare professional can thus anticipate the decompensation and initiate appropriate measures outside the emergency setting. An intermediate analysis is planned after the first 30 patients, possibly to set up a coordination cell with a nurse, as part of a delegation of tasks, as in TIM-HF2 [43]. Medical data can likewise be shared among health professionals, being part of a city-hospital network. Ultimately, an improvement in the patients' quality of life is to be expected.

DIABETe does not compete with Diabeo™ or other expert systems aimed at optimizing the glycemic balance, which is per se the main objective of diabetes management [41]. The DIABETe project focuses on the "global" management of diabetic patients through the detection of situations at risk of hospitalization: infection, cardiac decompensation, diabetic foot, as well as hypoglycemia and hyperglycemia episodes, potentially leading to hospitalizations [29, 42]. Regarding the remote monitoring platform used in DIABETe, an integration of or interfacing with expert systems such as Diabeo™ [41, 42] appears possible.

5. Perspectives regarding new developments in telemedicine

In the future, telemedicine projects will have to address some of today's medical issues (challenge for "tomorrow telemedicine") [29, 30]. Thus, the new solutions of telemedicine have to take into account the coexistence in the same individual of numerous chronic pathologies (e.g., diabetes, CHF, chronic obstructive pulmonary disease, chronic renal failure, etc.) and comorbidities (high BP, dyslipidemia, etc.). They have to offer complete and "global" management, including both social and medical dimensions. They have to resolve the specificities of elderly patients: no appetite for new technologies and new uses and their main problems (e.g., falls, malnutrition, mild cognitive impairment, etc.).

In this setting, the new developments in telemedicine are also to resolve the multiplicity of health professionals working with the same patient and the multiplicity of medical organizations (e.g., with or without human resources, telemedical center, etc.) [29, 30]. Today, the logistical obstacles to the implementation of

Overall mortality	Therapeutic education
Specific mortality of the considered chronic disease	Hygiene-dietary and therapeutic compliance
Number of hospitalization for the considered chronic disease	Optimization of food and sports hygiene
	Patient self-management
Number of re-hospitalization for the considered chronic disease	Optimization of the care pathway for the considered chronic disease
Number of hospitalization days	Structuring of the care pathway for the considered chronic disease
Health costs	
Management costs for the considered chronic disease	City-hospital relations
Number of days off work	Information sharing among health professionals
Quality of life	System use by health professionals

Table 2.
Potential parameters to be evaluated in a telemedicine project for chronic disease management.

telehealth are significant, as many health systems are not yet designed to integrate these technologies into existing information systems. It is therefore necessary to plan now for an interfacing of computer systems and the integration of future telemedicine solutions.

Considering the current problems of access to healthcare professionals, the new telemedicine solutions must be able to structure the patients' care pathways, a major medical topic that should interest our governments and authorities [28, 29]. Likewise, the E-care and DIABETe projects provide a means for healthcare professionals to exchange with each other, thereby facilitating patient access to medical resources. In this context, future research must also focus on the accessibility and practicality of telemedicine interventions.

Importantly, reimbursement remains a major concern and a barrier ("glass ceiling"). In fact, the healthcare delivered by telehealth is not covered by traditional fee-for-service payment models (e.g., in France, where all diabetic patients benefit from an integral treatment of their health expenses) [29]. The growth of value-based payment models may, however, provide incentives to implement telehealth as a strategy to provide high-quality, cost-effective, and coordinated care [29]. At country levels, variations in practice laws, restrictions on how telehealth can be delivered, and which patients should receive these services limit telemedicine's applicability as well [30].

Thus, to document the efficacy on the new telemedicine solutions, the future studies should integrate others objectives like potential targets to meet the needs and requirements of our societies, as listed in **Table 2**.

6. Conclusions

This review supports the efficacy of telemonitoring type 1 and type 2 diabetic patients. Several studies on diabetes telemonitoring, using diverse technologies, and transmitting different clinical, medical, and behavioral data were found. Significant impacts were observed, namely, at the behavioral, clinical, and structural levels. Minimal technical problems and cost-effectiveness analyses were reported. Four studies are dedicated specifically to elderly diabetic patients (all including <80-year-old patients).

Close management of diabetic patients, even elderly patients, through telemonitoring, showed the following: improvements in control of BG level and significant reduction in HbA1c, better appropriation of the disease by patients, greater adherence to therapeutic and hygiene-dietary measures, positive impact on comorbidities (arterial hypertension, weight, dyslipidemia), better patient's quality of life, and, at least, good receptiveness by patients and patient empowerment. Moreover, a cost-effectiveness analysis found a potential in medical economy. To date, the magnitude of its effects remains debatable, especially with the variation in patients' characteristics (e.g., background, ability for self-management, medical condition), sample selection, and approach for treatment of control groups.

To date, relatively few projects and trials in diabetic patients have been run within the "telemedicine 2.0" setting, using AI, ICT, and the Web 2.0. All these projects include real-life elderly diabetic patients. In this setting, it is the case of the project DIABETe. This project, as other projects listed in this review, is perfectly compatible with the care pathways being developed in chronic diseases by the authorities of industrialized countries, such as diabetes, chronic heart failure, and chronic obstructive pulmonary disease.

Further investigation of telemonitoring efficacy and cost-effectiveness over longer periods of time and larger samples is needed. Assessment of the attitude of providers is also important considering their heavy workload and issues of reimbursement.

Funding

Grants from the Fondation de l'Avenir, the Agence Régionale de Santé du Grand-Est (ARS) and the Agence Nationale de la Recherche (ANR).

Consent and Ethical approval

Not applicable.

Competing interest

M. Hajjam is the scientific director of *Predimed Technology* (www.predimed-technology.fr). All other authors have declared that no competing interests exist.

Ethical approval

Not applicable.

Guarantor

EA.

Contributorship

EA, LM and MH designed the paper and conducted the literature searches. EA, LM, AAZ, and MH drafted the results and parts of the discussion. ST, JD, JH, NJ, and AEHH provided critical analysis, revised the whole manuscript, and approved the final version for publication. EA is responsible for all revisions and remains in contact with the rest of the review team regarding status reports.

Author details

Emmanuel Andrès[1,2]*, Laurent Meyer[3], Abrar-Ahmad Zulfiqar[2,4], Mohamed Hajjam[5], Samy Talha[2,6], Sylvie Ervé[7], Jawad Hajjam[7], Nathalie Jeandidier[3] and Amir Hajjam El Hassani[8]

1 Service de Médecine Interne, Diabète et Maladies Métaboliques de la Clinique Médicale B, Hôpitaux Universitaires de Strasbourg, Strasbourg, France

2 Equipe de recherche EA 3072 "Mitochondrie, Stress oxydant et Protection musculaire", Faculté de Médecine de Strasbourg, Université de Strasbourg (Unistra), Strasbourg, France

3 Service d'Endocrinologie et de Diabétologie de la Clinique Médicale B, Hôpitaux Universitaires de Strasbourg, Strasbourg, France

4 Service de Médecine Interne, Gériatrie et Thérapeutique, CHU de Rouen, France

5 Predimed Technology, Strasbourg, France

6 Service de Physiologie et d'Explorations Fonctionnelles, Hôpitaux Universitaires de Strasbourg, Strasbourg, France

7 Centre d'expertise des Technologies de l'Information et de la Communication pour l'autonomie (CENTICH) et Mutualité Française Anjou-Mayenne (MFAM), Angers, France

8 Equipe de recherche EA 4662 "Nanomédecine, Imagerie, Thérapeutiques", Université de Technologie de Belfort-Montbéliard (UTBM), Belfort-Montbéliard, France

*Address all correspondence to: emmanuel.andres@chru-strasbourg.fr

References

[1] Haw JS, Galaviz KI, Straus AN, et al. Long-term sustainability of diabetes prevention approaches: A systematic review and meta-analysis of randomized clinical trials. JAMA Internal Medicine. 2017;**177**:1808-1817

[2] Nathan DM. Diabetes: Advances in diagnosis and treatment. JAMA. 2015;**314**:1052-1062

[3] Ostling Wyckoff J, Ciarkowski SL, et al. The relationship between diabetes mellitus and 30-day readmission rates. Clinical Diabetes and Endocrinology. 2017;**3**:3. DOI: 10.1186/s40842-016-0040-x

[4] Sinclair A, Dunning T, Rodriguez-Mañas L. Diabetes in older people: New insights and remaining challenges. The Lancet Diabetes and Endocrinology. 2015;**3**:275-285

[5] Ismail-Beigi F. Clinical practice. Glycemic management of type 2 diabetes mellitus. The New England Journal of Medicine. 2012;**366**:1319-1327

[6] Billiard A, Rohmer V, Roques MA, et al. Telematic transmission of computerized blood glucose profiles for IDDM patients. Diabetes Care. 1991;**14**:130-134

[7] Marrero DG, Vandagriff JL, Kronz K, et al. Using telecommunication technology to manage children with diabetes: The Computer-Linked Outpatient Clinic (CLOC) study. The Diabetes Educator. 1995;**21**:313-319

[8] Ahring KK, Ahring JP, Joyce C, et al. Telephone modem access improves diabetes control in those with insulin-requiring diabetes. Diabetes Care. 1992;**15**:971-975

[9] Liesenfeld B, Renner R, Neese M, et al. Telemedical care reduces hypoglycemias and improves glycemic control in children and adolescents with type 1 diabetes. Diabetes Technology & Therapeutics. 2000;**2**:561-567

[10] Bellazzi R, Larizza C, Montani S, et al. A telemedicine support for diabetes management: The T-IDDM project. Computer Methods and Programs in Biomedicine. 2002;**69**:147-161

[11] Biermann E, Dietrich W, Rihl J, et al. Is there time and cost savings by using telemanagement for patients on intensified insulin therapy? A randomized, controlled trial. Computer Methods and Programs in Biomedicine. 2002;**69**:137-146

[12] Welch G, Sokolove M, Mullin C, et al. Use of modem equipped blood glucose meter augmented with biweekly educator telephone support lowers HbA1c in type 1 diabetes. Diabetes. 2003;**52**(Suppl 1):A100

[13] Chase HP, Roberts MD, Pearson JA, et al. Modem transmission of glucose values reduces the costs and need for clinic visits. Diabetes Care. 2003;**26**:1475-1479

[14] Montori VM, Helgemoe PK, Guyatt GH, et al. Telecare for patients with type 1 diabetes and inadequate glycemic control: A randomized controlled trial and meta-analysis. Diabetes Care. 2004;**27**:1088-1094

[15] Vahatalo MA, Virtamo HE, Viikari JS, et al. Cellular phone transferred self-blood glucose monitoring: Prerequisites for positive outcome. Practical Diabetes International. 2004;**21**:192-194

[16] Bergenstal RM, Anderson RL, Bina DM, et al. Impact of modem-transferred blood glucose data on clinician work efficiency and patient glycemic control. Diabetes Technology & Therapeutics. 2005;**7**:241-247

[17] McMahon GT, Hu TMJ, Gomes HE, et al. Web-based care management in poorly controlled diabetes. Diabetes Care. 2005;**28**:1624-1629

[18] Farmer AJ, Hayton PM, Gibson OJ, et al. A randomized controlled trial of the effect of real-time telemedicine support on glycemic control in young adults with type 1 diabetes. Diabetes Care. 2005;**28**:2697-2702

[19] Cho JH, Song KH, Chang SA, et al. Long-term effect of the Internet-based glucose monitoring system on HbA1c reduction and glucose stability. Diabetes Care. 2006;**29**:2625-2631

[20] Gay CL, Chapuis F, Bendelac N, et al. Reinforced follow-up for children and adolescents with type 1 diabetes and inadequate glycemic control: A randomized controlled trial intervention via the local pharmacist and telecare. Diabetes & Metabolism. 2006;**32**:159-165

[21] Shea S, Weinstock RS, Starren J, et al. A randomized trial comparing telemedicine case management with usual care in older, ethnically diverse, medically underserved patients with diabetes mellitus. Journal of the American Medical Informatics Association. 2006;**13**:40-51

[22] Benhamou PY, Melki V, Boizel R, et al. One-year efficacy and safety of web-based follow-up using cellular phone in type 1 diabetic patients under insulin pump therapy: The PumpNet study. Diabetes & Metabolism. 2007;**33**:220-226

[23] Cadario F, Binotti M, Brustia M, et al. Telecare for teenagers with type 1 diabetes: A trial. Minerva Pediatrica. 2007;**59**:299-305

[24] Quinn CC, Clough SS, Minor JM, et al. WellDoc mobile diabetes management randomized controlled trial: Change in clinical and behavioral outcomes and patient and physician satisfaction. Diabetes Technology & Therapeutics. 2008;**10**:160-168

[25] McCarrier KP, Ralston JD, Hirsch IB, et al. Web-based collaborative care for type 1 diabetes: A pilot randomized trial. Diabetes Technology & Therapeutics. 2009;**11**:211-217

[26] Ralston JD, Hirsch IB, Hoath J, et al. Web-based collaborative care for type 2 diabetes: A pilot randomized trial. Diabetes Care. 2009;**32**:234-239

[27] Shea S, Weinstock RS, Teresi JA, et al. A randomized trial comparing telemedicine care management with usual care in older, ethnically diverse, medically underserved patients with diabetes mellitus: 5 year results of the IDEATel study. Journal of the American Medical Informatics Association. 2009;**16**:446-456

[28] https://www.legifrance.gouv.fr/eli/arrete/2017/4/25/AFSH1711560A/jo/texte/fr [November 2018]

[29] Andrès E, Hajjam M, Talha S, et al. Télémédecine dans le domaine de l'insuffisance cardiaque. État des lieux et focus sur le projet de télémédecine 2.0 E-care. Perspectives dans le domaine de la diabétologie. Médecine des Maladies Métaboliques. 2018;**12**:224-231

[30] Puricel SG, Ruiz J. Le diabète et l'ère de la télémédecine. Revue Médicale Suisse. 2014;**10**:1246-1248

[31] Ponikowski P, Voors AA, Anker SD, et al. 2016 ESC Guidelines for the diagnosis and treatment of acute and chronic heart failure: The Task Force for the diagnosis and treatment of acute and chronic heart failure of the European Society of Cardiology (ESC) Developed with the special contribution of the Heart Failure Association (HFA) of the ESC. European Heart Journal. 2016;**37**:2129-2200

[32] Stone R, Rao H, Sevick M, et al. Active care management supported by home telemonitoring in Veterans with type 2 diabetes: The DiaTel randomized controlled trial. Diabetes Care. 2009;**33**:478-484

[33] Stone R, Sevick M, Rao H, et al. The diabetes telemonitoring study extension: An exploratory randomized comparison of alternative interventions to maintain glycemic control after withdrawal of diabetes home telemonitoring. Journal of the American Medical Informatics Association. 2012;**19**:973-979

[34] Shane-McWhorter LL, Petersen M, et al. The Utah remote monitoring project: Improving health care one patient at a time. Diabetes Technology & Therapeutics. 2014;**16**:653-660

[35] Nicolucci A, Cercone S, Chiriatti A, Muscas F, Gensini G, on behalf of the REMOTE Study Group. A randomized trial on home telemonitoring for the management of metabolic and cardiovascular risk in patients with type 2. Diabetes Diabetes Technology & Therapeutics. 2015;**17**:8-13

[36] Katalenich B, Shi L, Liu S, et al. Evaluation of a remote monitoring system for diabetes control. Clinical Therapeutics. 2015;**37**:1216-1225

[37] Wild SH, Hanley J, Lewis SC, et al. Supported telemonitoring and glycemic control in people with type 2 diabetes: The telescot diabetes pragmatic multicenter randomized controlled trial. PLoS Medicine. 2016l;**e1002098**:13

[38] Turnin MC, Schirr-Bonnans S, Martini J, et al. Educ@dom: Comparative study of the telemonitoring of patients with type 2 diabetes versus standard monitoring-study protocol for a randomized controlled study. Diabetology and Metabolic Syndrome. 2017;**9**:52

[39] Lindberg I, Torbjørnsen A, Söderberg S, Ribu L. Telemonitoring and health counseling for self-management support of patients with type 2 diabetes: A randomized controlled trial. JMIR Diabetes. 2017;**2**:e10

[40] Charpentier G, Benhamou PY, Dardari D, et al. The Diabeo software enabling individualized insulin dose adjustments combined with telemedicine support improves HbA1c in poorly controlled type 1 diabetic patients: A 6-month, randomized, open-label, parallel-group, multicenter trial (TeleDiab 1 Study). Diabetes Care. 2011;**34**:533-539

[41] Jeandidier N, Chaillous L, Franc S, et al. DIABEO app software and telemedicine versus usual follow-up in the treatment of diabetic patients: Protocol for the TELESAGE randomized controlled trial. JMIR Research Protocols. 2018;**7**:e66. DOI: 10.2196/resprot.9154

[42] Andrès E, Talha S, Jeandidier N, Meyer L, Hajjam M, Hajjam A. Telemedicine in chronic diseases: The time of maturity with telemedicine 2.0 in the setting of chronic heart failure and diabetes mellitus! Current Research in Diabetes & Obesity Journal. 2018;**6**:1-4

[43] Koehler F, Koehler K, Deckwart O, Prescher S, Wegscheider K, Kirwan BA, et al. Efficacy of telemedical interventional management in patients with heart failure (TIM-HF2): A randomised, controlled, parallel-group, unmasked trial. Lancet. 2018;**392**:1047-1057

[44] Van De Belt TH, Engelen L, Berben S, Schoonhoven L. Definition of health 2.0 and medicine 2.0: A systematic review. Journal of Medical Internet Research. 2010;**12**:e18

[45] Benyahia A, Hajjam A, Andrès E, Hajjam M, Hilaire V. Including other system in E-Care telemonitoring

platform. Studies in Health Technology and Informatics. 2013;**190**:115-117

[46] Rjeily CB, Badr G, El Hassani AH, Andrès E. Medical data mining for heart diseases and the future of sequential mining. Machine Learning Paradigms: Advances in Data Analytics. 2018;**149**:71-99

[47] Andrès E, Talha S, Hajjam M, Hajjam J, Ervé S, Hajjam A. Experimentation of 2.0 telemedicine in elderly patients with chronic heart failure: A study prospective in 175 patients. European Journal of Internal Medicine. 2018;**51**:e11-e12

[48] Andrès E, Talha S, Benyahia AA, et al. e-Health: A promising solution for the optimized management of chronic diseases. Example of a national e-Health project E-care based on a e-plateform in the context of chronic heart failure. European Research in Telemedicine/La Recherche Européenne en Télémédecine. 2015;**4**:87-94

Chapter 6

Future Treatment of Alzheimer Disease

Ahmet Onur Keskin, Nazlı Durmaz, Gülgün Uncu, Ebru Erzurumluoglu, Zerrin Yıldırım, Nese Tuncer and Demet Özbabalık Adapınar

Abstract

Alzheimer's disease is an age-related progressive neurodegenerative disorder. The two major neuropathologic hallmarks of Alzheimer's disease (AD) are extracellular Amyloid beta (Aβ) plaques and intracellular neurofibrillary tangles (NFTs). A number of additional pathogenic mechanisms, possibly overlapping with Aβ plaques and NFTs formation, have been described, including inflammation, oxidative damage, iron dysregulation, cholesterol metabolism. To date, only symptomatic treatments exist for this disease, all trying to counterbalance the neurotransmitter disturbance. To block the progression of the disease they have to interfere with the pathogenic steps responsible for the clinical symptoms, including the deposition of extracellular amyloid β plaques and intracellular neurofibrillary tangle formation, inflammation and stem cell. In this review, we discuss new potential disease-modifying therapies for AD that are currently being studied in phase I–III trials.

Keywords: Alzheimer, secretase modulators, anti-amyloid agents, stem cell

1. Introduction

Alzheimer's disease (AD) is an age-related progressive neurodegenerative disorder characterized by progressive memory loss, cognitive impairment and functional decline. AD is described as a multifactorial disease and several mechanisms significant roles in disease pathogenesis. Through an improved understanding of the molecular mechanisms underlying pathogenesis of AD, it is possible to develop novel, effective therapeutic methods in order to prevent onset and progression of AD. A better understanding of the molecular mechanisms underlying pathogenesis of AD makes available to a basis for development of novel, effective therapeutic strategies to prevent onset and progression of AD.

The formation of intracellular neurofibrillary tangles that are composed of hyperphosphorylated tau proteins [1] and accumulation of extracellular amyloid plaques are the fundamental neuropathological changes noticed in AD brain. Aβ and tau are two key/important proteins, have a main function in the pathogenesis of AD. Amyloid cascade hypothesis and tau hypothesis have been based on the causative factors in AD pathogenesis. While one of these hypothesis proposes that AD starts with the accumulation of Aβ, the other one suggests that AD starts with the accumulation of p-tau.

Amyloid cascade hypothesis: in 1992 Hardy and Higgins constructed the amyloid-cascade hypothesis [2]. According to this hypothesis, formation of pathological Aβ plaques, neurofibrillary tangles, synaptic loss, neurodegeneration and ultimately dementia in AD are caused by a cascade harming synapses and neurons has been triggered by Aβ and its aggregates. Aβ peptides are natural products of brain metabolism. AD is associated with the disruption of the balance between production and clearance of Aβ. Aβ accumulation in the brain induces oxidative stress and inflammatory response thus leads to neurotoxicity which contributes to impairment of cognitive functions. Several pathological events like excitotoxicity, synaptic and mitochondrial dysfunction, loss of calcium homeostasis, endoplasmic reticulum stress, oxidative stress and inflammation may occur as a result of Aβ aggregates. In spite of the role of Aβ in AD, only amyloid-cascade hypothesis is not sufficient to explain AD pathogenesis, because removal of Aβ did not halt AD pathology [3].

Tau hypothesis: tau is an intracellular protein which is a member of microtubule-associated proteins family. This protein family promotes microtubule assembly and stabilization. Tau has neurotoxic effects when hyperphosphorylated due to loss of its normal function. Hyperphosphorylated tau promotes the formation of paired helical filaments which would eventually evolve into NFTs, dystrophic neurites, and neuropil threads [4]. Abnormal hyperphosphorylation of tau is a component of neurofibrillary tangles that is a key player of neurodegeneration and has been isolated from AD brain in the 1990s [5].

Although both hypotheses suggest primal roles of Aβ and tau protein in AD pathogenesis, increasing evidence suggests that there may be a crosstalk between two pathologies. However, the mechanisms linking Aβ toxicity and tau hyperphosphorylation have not been exactly clarified yet.

2. Pathogenic mechanisms in Alzheimer's disease

2.1 Oxidative stress

Oxygen metabolism generates free radicals such as reactive nitrogen species (RNS) and reactive oxygen species (ROS) including superoxide anion and hydroxyl radical. One of the early changes observed in AD patients is increased oxidative damage. It has been shown that the percentages of 8-hydroxydeoxyguanosine (8OHdG) and 8-hydroxyguanosine (DNA and RNA oxidation markers), 4-hydroxynonenal, and F2-isoprostanes (lipid peroxidation markers), protein carbonyls and 3-nitrotyrosine (protein oxidation markers), and malondialdehyde (MDA), have been increased in AD brains [6]. Although the data is highly limited, oxidative stress may also influence hyperphosphorylation and polymerization of tau protein. Although oxidative stress has an important role in AD, it is still disputed whether it plays a causative role in the disease or secondary to the pathological changes observed in AD [7].

2.2 Neuroinflammation

Neuroinflammation is described as a process involving activation of natural immunity in the brain. The functions of neuroinflammation can be explained as protecting central nervous system from infectious insults, injury or diseases. Microglia are has a significant role in neuroinflammation. Transgenic animal models of AD have demonstrated that neuroinflammation is enhanced around amyloid plaques [8]. According to Bellucci et al. inflammation is the key player in the tauopathies for neurodegeneration [9]. It has been shown that production of enzymes

(COX-2) and proinflammatory cytokines (IL-1β) are boosted in tau-positive nerve cells in spinal cord and brainstem. Pursuant to these results of the research, neuroinflammation might be triggered through NFTs by activating microglia. It is found that suppression of neuroinflammation is related to improvements in behavioral and cognitive deficits in AD mouse models and is in harmony with decline in hyperphosphorylated tau and Aβ plaques in brain. It is efficient to treat with interleukin-1β (IL-1β) antibodies or anti-tumor necrosis factor-α (anti-TNF-α) in order to reduce the pathology in animal models of AD. It is noted that Aβ secretion and the expression and activity of β-secretase have been reduced by peroxisome proliferator-activated receptor-γ [PPAR-γ] agonists and nonsteroidal anti-inflammatory drugs [NSAIDs] [10]. It is suggested that suppression of neuroinflammation with NSAIDs rescues memory and cognitive decline. While retrospective epidemiological studies have proven that prolonged treatment with NSAIDs delays onset of AD when initiated early stage or before disease initiation, its effectiveness has not been demonstrated in neither mild nor moderate forms of AD [11].

2.3 Metal toxicity

Iron, zinc and copper are important elements for neuronal function. During the aging, these metal ions accumulate in the brain, consequently contribute to neurodegeneration. Zinc, copper and iron have been found to be accumulated within the core and periphery of senile plaques and these metals have been suggested to be involved in Aβ aggregation and oxidative damage. Metal chelation is a therapy based on binding and removing to metal ions. This therapy can provide an advantageous against oxidative stress in AD. Desferrioxamine and clioquinol are several examples of treatment methods with metal chelators. And these methods have caught some success in order to alter the progression of AD [12]. Therapeutic approaches focusing on the improvement of metal balance are one of the popular subjects of current researches in the field of AD.

2.4 Mitochondrial dysfunction

Mitochondrial dysfunction has a significant function in brain aging and AD. Swerdlow and Kan suggested mitochondrial cascade hypothesis for sporadic form of AD in 2004 [13]. This hypothesis proposes that mitochondrial dysfunction exists early in disease pathogenesis and causes, NFT formation, Aβ deposition and synaptic loss, the mitochondria is vulnerable to oxidative stress because of lack of DNA repair activity and is the significant source of ROS in the central nervous system. Oxidation of mitochondrial DNA presents it vulnerable to somatic mutations which augments mitochondrial dysfunction. Mitochondrial dysfunction has been proposed to trigger onset of neuronal degeneration in AD. It is showed that Aβ accumulates in mitochondria from AD patients. Tau protein might also be included in mitochondrial dysfunction in synapse, indirectly.

2.5 Brain insulin resistance and insulin deficiency

Type 2 diabetes mellitus is a risk factor for AD and these two disorders share many common pathological pathways. Impaired glucose metabolism is related to rising oxidative stress and accumulated advanced glycation end products. Insulin is even produced in brain tissue itself. Insulin receptors are mostly located in the cerebral cortex, cerebellum, hypothalamus, hippocampus and olfactory bulb that are the cognition pertinent areas of the brain. Brain glucose utilization and insulin signaling are impaired in AD. AD is related to a reduction in the levels of insulin in the cerebrospinal fluid (CSF), in the ratio of CSF insulin/plasma insulin, a decline in the expression of insulin receptors and a rise in fasting plasma insulin levels. Impaired insulin signaling might influence AD pathogenesis via tau hyperphosphorylation, acetylcholine signaling and Aβ metabolism. Insulin stimulates the expression of choline acetyltransferase, the enzyme responsible for acetylcholine synthesis. Therefore, decreased insulin levels, as well as insulin resistance, can ultimately contribute to a decrease in acetylcholine in AD brains [14].

2.6 Future therapeutic approaches and management of AD

Alzheimer's disease [AD] is one of the most challenging threats to the healthcare system. The current therapeutic goals are to reduce amyloid levels, prevention of amyloid aggregation/toxicity and tau phosphorylation/aggregation. There is also a major improvement in understanding the role of cholinesterase [ChE] in the brain and the function of ChE inhibitors in AD Academic research has carried out on the system of a new generation of acetyl- and butyryl ChE inhibitors and test for AD in clinical experiments on human beings. Next to this alternative strategies for treating or slowing the progression of AD, like vaccination, anti-inflammatory agents, cholesterol-lowering agents, antioxidants and hormone therapy, are also studied. Although several anti-amyloid β compounds have been examined in clinical trials as potentially useful drugs, all of them have failed to show significant benefits so far. Tau-targeted drugs have been developed and have entered clinical trials recently. The improvements on early diagnostic biochemical markers will be useful to increase for better monitoring the course of the disease and to evaluate different therapeutic strategies [15].

Academic research of Alzheimer's disease consists three steps. The first one is to select a high-risk population with current evidence and to provide this population primary prevention. The goal of this first stage is to be able to manage modifiable risk factors. Second is to diagnose patients at the preclinical phase, which starts 10–20 years before symptoms occur. Researchers aim to find new and improve existing neuroimaging techniques, CSF investigations and laboratory and genetic studies. The third step is to discover disease-modifying molecules. Researchers are aiming to inhibit extracellular amyloid plaque accumulation and to inhibit intracellular tau-based neurofibrillary tangles accumulation [16].

2.6.1 Anti-amyloid agents

One of the main suggested pathophysiological processes is 'amyloid cascade hypothesis'. All autosomal dominant AD genetic forms are the result of mutations of amyloid metabolism encoding genes. Also clinical and experimental data indicates toxic effects of accumulated amyloid plaques. Amyloid directed therapies can be classified in three different classes: amyloid anti-aggregates, secretase modulators and immunotherapies [17].

2.6.2 Secretase modulators

To reduce Aβ production, researchers focused on modulate enzymes that breakdown amyloid precursor protein [by stimulating α secretase or inhibiting γ and β secretase activity]. While effective α secretase was infrequently, various γ and β secretase inhibitors improved. γ secretase plays a decisive role in Aβ generation but this enzyme has several cleavage actions including notch receptor signaling so that γ secretase inhibitors have significant side effects. β secretase inhibitors also failed to show disease-modifying effects but there are still ongoing studies [17].

2.6.3 Amyloid anti-aggregates

Another strategy is to prevent aggregation of amyloid in non-soluble forms. Although new studies report soluble form of Aβ also have toxic effects. It's known that Aβ forms oligomers, fibrils and then deposition of amyloid plaques exist. Tramiprosate, colostrinin, clioquinol are some of the studied anti-Aβ aggregation agents. There were no effects or minimal effects phase II and III anti-Aβ aggregation agents trials on cognition. There are ongoing projects to improve new molecules [18].

2.6.4 Amyloid removal [immunotherapy]

Although it is not proven (exactly) how immunotherapy might attenuate Aβ plaques in the brain, some mechanisms have postulated. Therapeutic goal is to induce a humoral immune response to fibrillary-Aβ42 or passive administration of anti-Aβ antibodies. First studies of active vaccination were halted because of the induction of serious side effects. There are ongoing phase I–III studies with active and passive immunization (CAD106, bapineuzumab, solanezumab, intravenous immunoglobulin) [18].

2.6.5 Tau-based therapies

Tau is a microtubule-associated protein and the MAPT gene encodes tau. Assembling microtubules and regulating axonal transport are various functions of tau. It is proven that hyperphosphorylated tau causes disruption of mitochondrial respiration and axonal transport. It should be emphasized that tau hyperphosphorylation is also considered as a pathologic sign of other neurodegenerative diseases, including, frontotemporal dementia with parkinsonism (FTD-P), corticobasal degeneration, progressive supranuclear palsy and Pick disease. Mutations of tau encoded MAPT1 gene causes FTD-P. Therefore neurodegeneration without amyloid deposition can be driven by tau dysfunction. Tau-based therapies are still at conceptual stages and include passive immunization against tau, preventing tau hyperphosphorylation and anti-aggregates of tau. Methylthioninium chloride and lithium are some of the elements with current studies. There are also some experiments ongoing about anti-tau vaccines at AD [19].

3. Treatments that failed in clinical trials

Only four cholinesterase inhibitors (tacrine, donepezil, rivastigmine, galantamine) and an *N*-methyl-D-aspartate (NMDA) receptor AD antagonist (memantine) are approved for the treatment of AD. These five drugs are all symptomatic treatments. No new drugs have been approved for treatment of AD since 2003. Disease modifying drugs (DMD) is the real goal in AD treatment. However, success rate is extremely low for Alzheimer treatment research. Until today, anti-inflammatory (NSAİD, steroids), antioxidant (selenium, vitamin E), anti-ischemic (statin, aspirin), cholinergic (lecithin), nutrients (Omega-3, vitamins B, folic acid), monoclonal antibody (bapineuzumab, solanezumab) treatments have failed (**Table 1**). The overall failure rate was 99.6% (0.4% success) in the decade spanning from 2002 to 2012 [20]. Many explanations have been proposed for the failures of trials of DMD for AD, including starting therapies at the late phase of disease, wrong or nonspecific treatment targets, incorrect doses, the lack of homogeneity of individuals (genetic, ethical, temporal and medical grounds), nonspecific or blunt trial design [21, 22]. On the other hand, pathological changes may not correlated with cognitive deficits

Agent	Proposed mode of action	Reason	Reference
Ganstigmine	Acetylcholinesterase inhibitor	Side effects (headache, nausea, vomiting, anorexia)	Racchi et al. [23]
Metrifonate	Cholinesterase inhibition (irreversible)	Side effects (neuromuscular dysfunction, respiratory failure)	Arrieta et al. [24]
Lecithin	Major dietary source of choline	There is no significant benefit of lecithin for Alzheimer's disease or Parkinsonian dementia	Higgins and Flicker [25]
Ibuprofen	Anti-inflammatory, NSAİD	No evidence yet exists ibuprofen is efficacious in Alzheimer's disease	Tabet and Feldman [26]
Rofecoxib	Cyclo-oxygenase-2 inhibition	No significant differences between treatments were found for the ADAS-cog score	Reines et al. [27]
Aspirin, steroid	Anti-inflammatory	No significant improvement in cognitive decline for aspirin and steroid	Jaturapatporn et al. [28]
Latrepirdine	Antihistamine drug	There is no effect of latrepirdine on cognition and function in mild-to-moderate AD patients	Chau et al. [29]
Selegiline	Monamine oxidase inhibition	The evidence of benefit using standardised global cognitive scales was extremely limited. There is not yet enough evidence to recommend its use in practice	Birks and Flicker [30]
Pravastatin	Lowers plasma cholesterol and lipoprotein	Pravastatin had no significant effect on cognitive function or disability	Shepherd [31]
Simvastatin, pravastatin	Lowers plasma cholesterol and lipoprotein	There is no evidence that statins prevent cognitive decline or dementia	McGuinness et al. [32]
Omega-3 polyunsaturated fatty acids	Essential dietary nutrient	There is not convincing evidence for the efficacy of omega-3 PUFA supplements in the treatment of mild to moderate AD	Burckhardt et al. [33]
Vitamin E, selenium	Antioxidant supplement	Antioxidant supplements did not prevent dementia	Kryscio et al. [34]
Vitamin E	Vitamin E, selenium	There is no evidence that vitamin E prevents dementia, or that it improves cognitive function in people with MCI or AD	Farina et al. [35]
Vitamins B	Methionine-synthase mediated conversion of homocysteine to methionine, antioxidant, nerve growth and repair	There is no adequate evidence of an effect of vitamins B on general cognitive function, executive function	Li et al. [36]
Acetyl-L-carnitine	Activity at cholinergic neurons, membrane stabilization and enhancing mitochondrial function	There is no evidence of benefit of improvement in cognition or functional ability	Hudson [37]

Agent	Proposed mode of action	Reason	Reference
Piracetam	Multiple complex mechanisms	The evidence does not support the use of piracetam in the treatment of people with dementia or cognitive impairment	Flicker and Evans [38]
Semagacestat	γ-Secretase inhibition	Serious adverse events (weight loss, skin cancers and infections), worsening of cognition and functioning	Doody et al. [39]
Tarenflurbil(R-flurbiprofen)	γ-Secretase inhibition	No effect on cognitive decline or the loss of daily living activities in mild AD	Green et al. [40]
Bapineuzumab	Humanized, N-terminal specific anti-Aβ monoclonal antibody	No significant improvement in cognition, serious side effects, vasogenic edema	Abushouk et al. [41]
Solanezumab	Humanized monoclonal IgG1 antibody directed against the mid-domain of the Aβ peptide	No significant improvement in cognition	Honig et al. [42]

Table 1.
The anti-AD drug candidates for which the clinical trials have been failed or suspended.

in AD, measuring cognitive abilities is a reductionist approach as the disease is too complex and transgenic animal models are not capable of mimicking the various pathophysiological mechanisms in humans. Several new chemical entities claiming to have potential benefits in AD have been developed by researchers all over the globe. However, the evolution of a definite disease modifying therapy for AD is constantly under the threat of chasing the wrong pathology [22].

4. Ongoing clinical trials for Alzheimer's disease

Alzheimer's disease (AD) is a neurodegenerative disorder resulting from progressive pathological changes characterized by protein deposits in the form of amyloid plaques (APs) and neurofibrillary tangles (NFTs), which cause synaptic and neuronal loss. According to generally accepted hypothesis AD starts with abnormal processing of amyloid precursor protein (APP) [2]. Excess production or reduced clearance of β-amyloid peptide monomers, which is produced by the amyloidogenic cleavage of the membrane-spanning protein APP are the two main mechanisms of this abnormal deposition process, which causes aggregation of β-amyloid (Aβ) fibrils in extracellular APs. Second core pathophysiological mechanism of the disease is the intraneuronal deposition of hyperphosphorylated tau (pT) within NFTs [5].

Synaptic dysfunction, mitochondrial and oxidative changes, neuroinflammation, gliosis, and finally apoptosis and neuronal loss are known neurodegenerative consequences of AD, which are reflected in the macroscopical level as the regional cortical atrophy starting from limbic regions of the brain and then traveling trans synaptically to paralimbic, heteromodal and finally to unimodal association cortices. These changes and dysfunctions of the neurotransmitter systems such as acetylcholine, serotonin, glutamate, noradrenaline, dopamine cause clinical manifestations.

All these pathological changes are the targets of ongoing clinical trials for the treatment of AD. The term "disease-modifying strategies in AD" primarily connotes treatment strategies aiming at the prevention of and/or clearance of pathological Aβ and tau. Neurotransmitter-based strategies and others, such as combatting against oxidative stress or neuroinflammation are generally classified as "symptomatic treatments". In this section, current disease-modifying and symptomatic treatment strategies will be reviewed.

4.1 Amyloid-focused ongoing clinical trials

According to the amyloid cascade hypothesis, AD begins with the accumulation of Aβ, years before its clinical onset. APP is a transmembrane protein whose physiological function is not completely understood. In a healthy brain, APP is metabolized by three proteolytic enzymes, namely α, β and γ secretases [43]. Proximally, γ-secretase cleaves the protein in its membrane-spanning domain solely by itself, forming an intracellular carboxy-terminal fragment (CTF), which is probably pro-plastic by translocating into the neuronal nucleus and playing a role in pro-plastic signaling. However distally, APP is cleaved alternatively, either by α-secretase or by β-secretase (BACE) on its two different sites in the extracellular domain close to the amino terminal of APP. The former cleavage is non-amyloidogenic since it produces an inert peptide called p3 in the mid-segment and another one, which is called sAPPα containing the N-terminus and probably having some neurotrophic functions. However, the latter cleavage is amyloidogenic, since it produces the anti-plastic and deposition-prone Aβ fragment in the mid-segment and sAPPβ in the N-terminus. The resulting Aβ will either be cleared by lysosomal-proteasomal mechanisms or will oligomerize and start to induce its pathophysiological functions. Now it is known that soluble oligomers of Aβ are more toxic than its more downstream moieties that are insoluble protofibrils and fibrils [44, 45].

Therefore, current studies aim to agonize α-secretase activity (ADAM10 activators), inhibit β-secretase (BACE inhibitors), and inhibit or modulate γ-secretase (GSIs and GSMs). Also enhancing clearance of Aβ with active or passive immunotherapies or prevention of aggregation of APs are the treatment focuses of ongoing trials. Monoclonal antibodies bind different epitopes which are N-terminal, C-terminal or mid-domain of Aβ and different conformations of Aβ which are monomer, oligomer and fibril [46].

4.1.1 Reducing Aβ production

Two secretases, namely α and γ are seemingly no longer the focus of drug development efforts for AD, as a result of many failures in clinical trials and concerns that their interaction with other substrates may trigger diseases like cancer. Specific ADAM10 activators that will act only in the brain thus preventing its potential role in breast cancer is yet to be developed [47] In a recent review it was stated that "the future of γ-secretase inhibition as an AD treatment strategy may depend on the development of GSMs, which aim to cause a shift from Aβ1-42 species toward the shorter and less pathogenic forms of Aβ, while also sparing Notch" [48].

β-Secretase is an aspartic acid protease belongs to the pepsin family. β-Site APP cleaving enzyme 1 (BACE1) plays role in Aβ production. BACE1 inhibition strategies do not share the same concerns for interfering with the other secretases. Therefore BACE1 inhibition is one of the strategies to interfere with amyloid cascade. There are ongoing trials with E 2609 (NCT03036280, NCT02956486), CNP520 (NCT02565511, NCT03131453) and JNJ-54861911 (NCT02569398, NCT01760005) [49].

4.1.2 Aβ clearance

The first experience of active vaccine trial was with AN1792 and ended occurrence of T-cell mediated meningoencephalitis [50]. Now the only ongoing active vaccine trial is CAD-106 that generates anti-Aβ antibodies to N-terminus [51, 52].

Crenezumab is a humanized IgG4 monoclonal antibody (mAb) that binds the mid-domain of the Aβ peptide (residues 13–24) and binds multiple conformations of Aβ (monomers, oligomers, fibrils) [53, 54]. Patients with mild to moderate Alzheimer Disease and also Preclinical Presenilin1 (PSEN1) E280A Mutation Carriers are involved in ongoing trials of Crenezumab (NCT03491150, NCT03114657, NCT02353598, NCT01998841, NCT02670083).

Gantenerumab is a first fully human IgG1 mAb binds an N-terminal [3–12] and central [18–27] amino acids of the Aβ peptide. It binds monomers weaker than oligomers and fibrils [46]. Gantenerumab is being evaluated in phase 2 and 3 trials in individuals with prodromal and early AD and individuals at risk for and with early-stage autosomal-dominant AD (NCT02051608, NCT03444870, NCT03443973, NCT01224106, NCT01760005) [46, 55, 56].

Aducanumab is a fully human IgG1 mAb binds the N-terminus (residues 3–6) of Aβ peptide. It recognizes oligomers and fibrils but it does not react to the monomers [18]. Ongoing Aducanumab trials involve prodromal, early and mild AD patients (NCT03639987, NCT02484547, NCT02477800, NCT01677572) [46, 57].

Solanezumab is a humanized IgG1 mAb, binds the mid-domain of Aβ (residues 16–26). It specifically recognizes monomers [58]. There are two ongoing prevention trials with solanezumab (NCT01760005, NCT02008357).

4.1.3 Other anti-amyloidogenic compounds

In addition to abovementioned strategies, there are some other anti-amyloidogenic compounds with diverse mechanisms. ALZT-OP1 prevents Aβ aggregation and neuroinflammation and is being evaluated in phase III clinical trial (NCT02547818) [59]. Posiphen is another anti-amyloidogenic drug that currently in phase I/II clinical trial (NCT02925650) [60].

Update of selected anti-Alzheimer's disease drugs in clinical trials including anti-amyloid strategies are summarized in **Table 2**.

4.2 Tau-focused ongoing clinical trials

Tau is a microtubule-associated protein (MAP) in neurons which regulates the axonal transport [63]. Although tau pathology proved to be more correlated with clinical symptoms than amyloid mechanisms, tau-based therapeutic strategies are relatively new. Beta-folded oligomers of abnormal phosphorylation of tau are the main component of NFTs. Post-translational modifications such as phosphorylation, acetylation and truncation play a major role in tau function [64]. Modulating tau phosphorylation, targeting other tau post-translational modifications, microtubule stabilizers, tau aggregation inhibitors, anti-tau immunotherapy are the mechanisms targeted by clinical trials. Current clinical trials focusing on tau are summarized in **Table 3**.

4.2.1 Targeting tau-post-translational modifications

Salsalate is a nonsteroidal anti-inflammatory drug that has been shown to inhibit acetyltransferase p300-induced tau acetylation in frontotemporal dementia (FTD) mouse model [75]. There is a phase I clinical trial in patients with prodromal to mild

Target	Drug name	Study title	Therapy type	Trial status	Company	Clinical trial identifier
BACE inhibitor	E2609 Elenbecestat [49]	A 24 Month Study to Evaluate the Efficacy and Safety of E2609 in Subjects with Early Alzheimer's Disease_ (MissionAD2)	Small molecule	Phase III	Biogen, Eisai Co., Ltd.	NCT03036280
		A 24-Month Study to Evaluate the Efficacy and Safety of E2609 in Subjects with Early Alzheimer's Disease_ (MissionAD2)	Small molecule	Phase III	Biogen, Eisai Co., Ltd.	NCT02956486
	CNP520 [49]	A Study of CAD106 and CNP520 Versus Placebo in Participants at Risk for the Onset of Clinical Symptoms of Alzheimer's Disease	Small molecule	Phase II/III	Amgen, Inc., Novartis Pharmaceuticals Corporation	NCT02565511
		A Study of CNP520 Versus Placebo in Participants at Risk for the Onset of Clinical Symptoms of Alzheimer's Disease	Small molecule	Phase II/III	Amgen, Inc., Novartis Pharmaceuticals Corporation	NCT03131453
	JNJ-54861911 [49]	An Efficacy and Safety Study of Atabecestat in Participants Who Are Asymptomatic at Risk for Developing Alzheimer's Dementia (EARLY)	Small molecule	Phase II/III	Janssen, Shionogi Pharma	NCT02569398
		Dominantly Inherited Alzheimer Network Trial: An Opportunity to Prevent Dementia. A Study of Potential Disease Modifying Treatments in Individuals at Risk for or With a Type of Early Onset Alzheimer's Disease Caused by a Genetic Mutation.	Small molecule	Phase II/III	Janssen, Shionogi Pharma	NCT01760005
Aβ clearance	CAD106 [49, 61]	A Study of CAD106 and CNP520 Versus Placebo in Participants at Risk for the Onset of Clinical Symptoms of Alzheimer's Disease	Active immunotherapy	Phase II/III	Novartis Pharmaceuticals Corporation	NCT02565511
	Crenezumab	An Open-Label Crenezumab Study in Patients with Alzheimer's Disease	Passive immunotherapy	Phase III	Hoffmann-La Roche	NCT03491150
		A Study of Crenezumab Versus Placebo to Evaluate the Efficacy and Safety in Participants with Prodromal to Mild Alzheimer's Disease (CREAD 2)		Phase III	Hoffmann-La Roche	NCT03114657

DOI: http://dx.doi.org/10.5772/intechopen.85096

Target	Drug name	Study title	Therapy type	Trial status	Company	Clinical trial identifier
		A Study of Crenezumab Versus Placebo in Preclinical Presenilin1 (PSEN1) E280A Mutation Carriers to Evaluate Efficacy and Safety in the Treatment of Autosomal-Dominant Alzheimer's Disease, Including a Placebo-Treated Non-Carrier Cohort [27]		Phase II	• Genentech, Inc. • Banner Alzheimer's Institute • National Institute on Aging (NIA)	NCT01998841
		CREAD Study: A Study of Crenezumab Versus Placebo to Evaluate the Efficacy and Safety in Participants with Prodromal to Mild Alzheimer's Disease [20]		Phase III	AC Immune SA, Genentech, Hoffmann-La Roche	NCT02670083
	Gantenerumab	A Study of Gantenerumab in Participants with Mild Alzheimer Disease	Passive immunotherapy	Phase III	Hoffmann-La Roche	NCT02051608
		A Study of Gantenerumab in Participants with Prodromal Alzheimer's Disease [56]		Phase III	Hoffmann-La Roche	NCT01224106
		Dominantly Inherited Alzheimer Network Trial: An Opportunity to Prevent Dementia. A Study of Potential Disease Modifying Treatments in Individuals at Risk for or With a Type of Early Onset Alzheimer's Disease Caused by a Genetic Mutation. (DIAN-TU) [55]		Phase II Phase III	• Washington University School of Medicine, Eli Lilly and Company, Hoffmann-La Roche (and 5 more)	NCT01760005
	Aducanumab	A Study of Aducanumab in Participants with Mild Cognitive Impairment Due to Alzheimer's Disease or With Mild Alzheimer's Disease Dementia to Evaluate the Safety of Continued Dosing in Participants with Asymptomatic Amyloid-Related Imaging Abnormalities	Passive immunotherapy (against aggregated Aβ)	Phase II	Biogen	NCT03639987
		221AD302 Phase 3 Study of Aducanumab (BIIB037) in Early Alzheimer's Disease (EMERGE) [46]		Phase III	Biogen	NCT02484547

Target	Drug name	Study title	Therapy type	Trial status	Company	Clinical trial identifier
		21AD301 Phase 3 Study of Aducanumab (BIIB037) in Early Alzheimer's Disease (ENGAGE) [46]		Phase III	Biogen	NCT02477800
		Multiple Dose Study of Aducanumab (BIIB037) (Recombinant, Fully Human Anti-Aβ IgG1 mAb) in Participants with Prodromal or Mild Alzheimer's Disease (PRIME) [57]		Phase I	Biogen	NCT01677572
	Solanezumab	Dominantly Inherited Alzheimer Network Trial: An Opportunity to Prevent Dementia. A Study of Potential Disease Modifying Treatments in Individuals at Risk for or With a Type of Early Onset Alzheimer's Disease Caused by a Genetic Mutation. (DIAN-TU) [55]	Passive immunotherapy (against Aβ3–12 and Aβ18–27)	Phase II Phase III	• Washington University School of Medicine • Eli Lilly and Company • Hoffmann-La Roche (and 5 more)	NCT01760005
		Clinical Trial of Solanezumab for Older Individuals Who May be at Risk for Memory Loss [62]		Phase III	• Eli Lilly and Company • Alzheimer's Therapeutic Research Institute	NCT02008357
Other Anti-amyloidogenic Compounds	ALZT-OP1 [59]	Safety and Efficacy Study of ALZT-OP1 in Subjects with Evidence of Early Alzheimer's Disease (COGNITE)		Phase III	AZTherapies, Inc.	NCT02547818
	Posiphen® [60]	Safety, Tolerability, PK and PD of Posiphen® in Subjects with Early Alzheimer's Disease (DISCOVER)		Phase I Phase II	• QR Pharma Inc. • Alzheimer's Disease Cooperative Study (ADCS)	NCT02925650

Table 2.
Update of selected anti-Alzheimer's disease drugs in clinical trials including anti-amyloid strategies.

Target	Drug name	Study title	Therapy type	Trial status	Company/sponsor	Clinical trial identifier
Lisin acetylation inhibitor	Salsalate [65]	Salsalate in Patients Mild to Moderate Alzheimer's Disease	Small molecule	Phase I	Adam Boxer	NCT03277573
c-Abl inhibitor	Nilotinib [66]	Impact of Nilotinib on Safety, Biomarkers and Clinical Outcomes in Mild to Moderate Alzheimer's Disease	c-Abl inhibitor	Phase II	Georgetown University	NCT02947893
Microtubule stabilizers	TPI-287	A Safety, Tolerability, Pharmacokinetics, Pharmacodynamics and Preliminary Efficacy Study of TPI-287 in Alzheimer's Disease	Small molecule	Phase I	Cortice Biosciences	NCT01966666
Tau aggregation inhibitors	TRX-0237 [67, 68]	Safety and Efficacy of TRx0237 in Subjects with Early Alzheimer's Disease	Small molecule	Phase II-III	• TauRx Therapeutics Ltd	NCT03446001
	Nicotinamide	Nicotinamide as an Early Alzheimer's Disease Treatment (NEAT)	Lysosomal acidification	Phase II	• University of California, Irvine	NCT03061474
Anti-Tau immunoteraphies	AADvac-1 [67]	24 Months Safety and Efficacy Study of AADvac1 in Patients with Mild Alzheimer's Disease	Active immunotherapy	Phase II	Axon Neuroscience SE	NCT02579252
	ACI-35 [19]	A study comparing the safety and effects of a new compound, ACI-35 with placebo in patients with mild to moderate Alzheimer's disease	Active immunotherapy	Phase I	AC Immune SA, Janssen	ISRCTN13033912
	IvIg [69–71]	Study of Intravenous Immunoglobulin in Amnestic Mild Cognitive Impairment	Active immunotherapy	Phase II	• Sutter Health	NCT01300728
		A Study to Evaluate Albumin and Immunoglobulin in Alzheimer's disease	Active immunotherapy	Phase II Phase III	Instituto Grifols, S.A./ Grifols Biologicals Inc.	NCT01561053
	ABBV-8E12 [72, 73]	A Study to Evaluate the Efficacy and Safety of ABBV-8E12 in Subjects with Early Alzheimer's Disease	Passive Immunotherapy	Phase II	AbbVie	NCT02880956
		An Extension Study of ABBV-8E12 in Early Alzheimer's Disease	Passive Immunotheraphy	Phase II	AbbVie	NCT03712787
	RO 7105705 [74]	A Study to Evaluate the Efficacy and Safety of RO7105705 in Patients with Prodromal to Mild Alzheimer's Disease	Passive Immunotheraphy	Phase II	Genentech, Inc	NCT03289143

Table 3.
Current clinical trials focusing on tau.

AD (NCT03277573). Nilotinib is a c-Abl tyrosine kinase inhibitor used in patients with leukemia [76]. It is thought to clean tau by inducing autophagy. It is being evaluated in a phase II clinical trial in patients with mild to moderate AD (NCT02947893).

4.2.2 Microtubule stabilizers

TPI-287 is a small molecule that stabilizes microtubules. It is tested in a phase I clinical trial in AD patients [77].

4.2.3 Tau aggregation inhibitors

LMT-X or named as TRx0237 is a second generation formulation of methylene blue that targets tau accumulation [77]. There is a phase II/III clinical trial in patients with early AD (NCT03446001) [67, 68]. Nicotinamide is the precursor of coenzyme Nicotinamide adenine dinucleotide prevents phosphorylation of tau in mice. A phase II study in mild-to-moderate Alzheimer's disease is currently ongoing (NCT03061474).

4.2.4 Active immunotherapy

There are three active immunotherapy agents being evaluated in ongoing trials. AADvac-1 contains synthetic tau peptide spanning residues 294–305 derived from a naturally occurring truncated and misfolded tau protein coupled to keyhole limpet hemocyanin and aluminum hydroxide as adjuvant [77]. A phase II clinical trial in subjects with mild AD is ongoing (NCT02579252) [78]. ACI-35 is a synthetic peptide spanning the human protein tau sequence 393–408, phosphorylated at S396 and S404 [72]. A phase I clinical trial in subjects with mild to moderate AD is ongoing (ISRCTN13033912) [19]. Intravenous immunoglobulin (IVIg) is a human plasma-derived product consisting of polyclonal serum IgG used as anti-inflammatory and immunomodulatory therapy for various neurological diseases [73]. There are phase II and III studies in subjects with mild cognitive impairment and AD (NCT01300728, NCT01561053) [69, 70].

4.2.5 Passive immunotherapy

ABBV-8E12 is a humanized anti-tau monoclonal antibody. There are two studies with ABBV-8E12 in patients with early AD (NCT02880956, NCT03712787) [72, 73]. Another passive immunotherapy agent R07105705 is an anti-tau antibody [39]. It is being evaluated in patients with prodromal to mild AD (NCT03289143) [74].

4.3 Other ongoing clinical trials

Riluzole, a sodium channel blocker, is used as a disease-modifying drug for amyotrophic lateral sclerosis [79]. It lowers extracellular glutamate levels, inhibits presynaptic glutamate release and induces glutamate transporter activity. Riluzole is being evaluated in a Phase II clinical trial in patients with mild AD (NCT01703117) [79–82].

LMA11A-31 is a small molecule prevents synaptic dysfunction, spine loss, neurite degeneration, microglial activation, and cognitive deficits in animal models [83, 84]. A phase I/II trial with mild to moderate AD patients is ongoing (NCT03069014) [85]. AD is thought to be linked with viral infections [86, 87]. Therefore a phase II trial is ongoing in mild AD patients who test positive for serum antibodies for herpes simplex virus 1 or 2, with valacyclovir (NCT03282916). Lifestyle interventions, management of metabolic and cardiovascular risk factors,

DOI: http://dx.doi.org/10.5772/intechopen.85096

Target	Drug name	Study title	Therapy type	Trial status	Company	Clinical trial identifier
Glutaminergic	Riluzole [79–82]	Riluzole in Mild Alzheimer's Disease	Small molecule	Phase II	Sanofi	NCT01703117
Neurotrophins and Their Receptor-based Therapies	LM11A-31-BHS [85]	Study of LM11A-31-BHS in Mild–moderate AD Patients		Phase I Phase II	• PharmatrophiX Inc. • National Institute on Aging (NIA)	NCT03069014
Therapies Targeted at Neuroinflammation and Oxidative Stress	Valacyclovir [85]	Anti-viral Therapy in Alzheimer's Disease		Phase II	New York State Psychiatric Institute National Institutes of Health (NIH) National Institute on Aging (NIA)	NCT03282916
Therapies and Interventions for AD Prevention	Insulin (Humulin R® U-100) [85]	The Study of Nasal Insulin in the Fight Against Forgetfulness (SNIFF)		Phase II Phase III		NCT01767909

Table 4.
Other strategies of Alzheimer's disease treatment.

exercise and diet are the focuses for primary prevention of AD (NCT01767909, NCT03249688) [88–92].

Deep brain stimulation is a novel therapeutic strategy for AD. One trial is ongoing in patients with mild AD (NCT03622905). Other strategies of Alzheimer's disease treatment are summarized in **Table 4**.

5. Gene and stem cell therapy in Alzheimer disease

5.1 Genetics of Alzheimer's disease

Both age and family history are important risk factors for AD. The risk of developing AD increases for one who has a first-degree relative with AD when compared to the general population. AD can be grouped into two subtypes with respect to age of onset. Most of the AD cases (>95%) are late-onset AD (sporadic/LOAD) (above age 65) that is considered to be multifactorial [93]. Many susceptibility genes for LOAD have been defined thanks to genome-wide association studies (GWAS) and several other sequencing analyzes. For instance, one of the well-studied genetic risk factors for LOAD is an alteration in Apolipoprotein E (APOE) coded by the gene localized to 19q13 [94]. APOE is a multifunctional protein which serves a number of functions in neuronal activities. In brain tissue, there are three main isoforms that are diversified by each other by different one amino acid, which are APOEε2 (Cys112, Cys158), APOEε3 (Cys112, Arg158) and APOEε4 (Arg112, Arg158). The differences between these three APOE isoforms have a significant impact on the structure and function of APOE at molecular and cellular levels. Therefore, those are thought as associated with neuropathological conditions [95].

Early onset AD (Familial/EOAD) represent <5% of all cases of AD. APP (Amyloid beta (A4) precursor protein), PSEN1 (Presenilin 1), and PSEN2 (Presenilin 2) genes mutations are exclusively considered as a basis for EOAD in most cases [94]. APP, a transmembrane protein in neuron cells, is cleaved by β-secretase and γ-secretase, respectively, to produce β-amyloids (Aβ) and some other side products [96]. Since neurotoxic consequences of altered Aβ ratios like neurodegeneration resulting from aberrant synaptic function take place in brain, APP mutations have continuously been investigated. Yet, only approximately 15% of EOAD could be enlightened by dominant APP gene mutations [97].

Another protein that is strictly associated with the progression of AD is PSEN1 as it is the principal component of γ-secretase complex. Since neurotoxic fragments are formed by proteolytic function of γ-secretase on APP, PSEN1 gene mutations give rise to abnormal activity of the proteolytic enzyme leading to abnormal or longer Aβ fragments and, therefore this contributes to development of EOAD [95]. More than 180 autosomal dominant PSEN1 mutations associated with AD have been reported, which makes PSEN1 significantly important protein in the occurrence of EOAD [98]. Disease-causing PSEN1 gene mutations, showing complete penetrance, accounts for majority of EOAD (approximately 80%) and these mutations are defined as the most common cause of the disease [99]. Lastly, the gene PSEN2 is also coding for one subunit of γ-secretase, the aspartyl protease generates Aβ. Missense mutations are reported in PSEN2, which are rarely genetic basis of EOAD [100]. In total, as mentioned in Zou's review article in 2013, majority of the disease-causing mutations identified for the EOAD have been reported in PSEN1 gene (approximately 78%), followed by APP mutations (17%) then with rare PSEN2 gene mutations (approximately 5%) [94].

Technological advances in sequencing methods over the past decade allow researchers to investigate AD thoroughly, especially genetic fundamentals of the disease. Since high-throughput sequencing provides a large number of polymorphisms in numerous subjects, new several genes associated with AD risk have been emerged and reported [96]. Accordingly, genome-wide association studies (GWAS) about AD increased, which consequently suggests new gene therapy strategies.

5.2 Gene therapy for AD

Discovering risk loci by GWAS studies may help to enlighten the biological mechanisms underlying AD because the reported genes might have been target for medicines, thereby this issue promises further investigation in order to improve gene therapy strategies and thus precision medicine concept for AD [101].

Over time, gene delivery of nerve growth factor (NGF), brain-derived neurotrophic factor (BDNF), APOE, ECE (endothelin-converting enzyme) have been investigated in several animal models of AD. Endothelin-converting enzyme (ECE) is protease involved in the degradation of Aβ peptides. Intracranial administration of five recombinant adeno-associated viral vector (rAAV) containing the ECE-1 synthetic gene showed reduced Aβ in the anterior cortex and hippocampus in APP-PS1 transgenic mice. Use of AAV vector encoding anti-Aβ Ab in Tg2576 mice results in a significant decrease in Aβ level in the brain of subjects. These results support its use for the prevention and treatment of AD [102].

The first clinical trial using Adeno-Associated Virus delivery of NGF has been accomplished and the results indicate amelioration of AD pathogenesis. Clinical trials were conducted using CERE-110 that is an AAV2/2 vector containing full length NGF transgene for the treatment of AD patients. These trials confirmed that AAV2-NGF delivery was well tolerated with a high level of safety and no systemic toxicity but did not affect clinical outcomes or selected AD biomarkers (NCT00087789, NCT00876863) [103].

5.3 Stem cell treatment for AD

Stem cells (SCs) are continuously capable of self-renewing and differentiating into specialized cells. Accordingly, SC therapy is surely becoming a promising strategy in the treatment of neurodegenerative diseases including AD owing to the capacity of SCs to migrate and reach areas of the brain. SCs are classified into four groups; embryonic stem cells (ESCs), induced pluripotent stem cells (iPSCs), mesenchymal stem cell, and neural stem cells [104].

5.3.1 Embryonic stem cells (ESCs)

ESCs, called as pluripotent, are derived from the inner cell mass of blastocyst because they have the ability to develop cell types from the ectoderm, mesoderm, and endoderm germ layers [105]. ESCs may an excellent cell replacement therapy approaches for transplantation in AD [104]. In vitro studies have been successful to differentiate ESCs into specific neuronal cell types like dopaminergic neurons and these studies show that the role of ESCs and their derivatives reduce AD pathology in rodent models [106, 107].

Several studies reveal that ESC-derived NSCs can be safely transplanted without tumorigenesis despite the fact that undifferentiated ESCs have risks of tumor formation, transplantation rejection and immune responses [106, 108, 109]. Experiments conducted on human ESCs have been able to generate dopaminergic neurons, spinal motor neurons and astroglial cells [110]. Some studies demonstrated use of retinoic acid (RA) induce direct differentiation of human ESCs into basal forebrain cholinergic neurons (BFCNs). Tang et al. showed that ESC-derived

NPC transplantation into an Aβ-injured rat model improves memory impairment compared to sham controls [106].

5.3.2 Induced pluripotent stem cells (IPSCs)

Induced pluripotent stem cells could be generated from adult cells by the overexpression of key transcription factors (OCT4, SOX2, KLF4, LIN28, and NANOG) [111, 112]. iPSCs are in general similar to embryonic stem cells (ESCs) in morphology, gene expression profile and potential of differentiation [113].

Human iPSCs derived from AD patients' somatic cells can provide a new perspective to develop new strategies for disease modeling. Yagi et al. showed that fAD-iPSC-derived differentiated neurons have increased amyloid β42 secretion, responds to γ-secretase inhibitors and modulators, indicating the potential for identification and validation of candidate drugs [114]. Takamatsu et al. used iPSCs to derive macrophage-like myeloid lineage cells that could express neprilysin which is a protease with Aβ-degrading activity [115].

Recent studies have shown reprogramming structural chromosomal abnormalities and aberrant DNA methylation patterns in hiPSCs [116]. iPSCs can be edited by gene editing technologies like recombinant homologous, transcription activator-like effector nucleases (TALENs), clustered regularly interspaced short palindromic repeats (CRISPR-cas9) and can function as more suitable for cell transplantation.

5.3.3 Mesenchymal stem cells (MSCs)

Mesenchymal stem cells (MSCs) are adult multipotent progenitors and can be obtained from various adult tissues including bone marrow, peripheral blood, umbilical cord, adipose tissue, amniotic fluid. MSCs are most favored cell types in the treatment of AD due to their accessibility, relative ease of handling, secretion of a wide range of cytokines, easily transplanted intravenously into patients, and lack of ethical issues.

Most important features of ESCs is a wide range of differentiation potentials including neuronal cells [110]. Park et al. reported that transplanted human adipose tissue derived mesenchymal stem cells (ADMSCs) differentiate into neural cells in the brain and these cells can restore cognitive functions of mice by increasing acetylcholine synthesis, brain-derived neurotrophic factor (BDNF), nerve growth factor (NGF) and restoring neuronal integrity [117]. In addition, MSC transplantation has been shown to inhibit Aβ and tau-related cell death, and to reduce Aβ residues and plaque formation by modulating neuroinflammation [118, 119]. It has been reported that bone marrow-derived mesenchymal stem cells provide a reduction in Aβ deposits and facilitate changes in key proteins required for synaptic transmissions such as dynamin 1 and synapsin 1 [120].

5.3.4 Neural stem cells (NSCs)

Transplantation of growth factor-secreting NSC was reported to increase neurogenesis and cognitive function in a rodent AD model [121]. And the overexpression of NSC derived cholinergic neurons restored cognitive performance and synaptic integrity in a rodent model [122].

6. Conclusion

Alzheimer's disease is a progressive neurodegenerative disease that affects the central nervous system. Many complex pathological and genetic features have been described in the disease. Aβ aggregation, tau aggregation, metal dyshomeostasis, oxidative stress, cholinergic dysfunction, inflammation and downregulation of autophagy based on pathophysiological changes occur during the onset and progression of AD have been proposed. There is no effective treatment currently, however, at present, current drug treatments of AD, such as cholinesterase inhibitors or NMDA antagonists, mainly help to manage symptoms hereby obviating the need for new approaches to deal with AD underlying mechanisms. Ongoing advances in the knowledge of pathogenesis, in the identification of novel targets, in improved outcome measures, and in identification and validation of biomarkers may lead to effective strategies for AD prevention.

Author details

Ahmet Onur Keskin[1], Nazlı Durmaz[2], Gülgün Uncu[3], Ebru Erzurumluoglu[4], Zerrin Yıldırım[5], Nese Tuncer[6] and Demet Özbabalık Adapınar[7]*

1 Neurology Department, Adana Hospital, Baskent University, Turkey

2 Neurology Department, Medical Faculty, Eskisehir Osmangazi University, Turkey

3 Neurology Department, Eskisehir City Hospital, Turkey

4 Medical Genetic Department, Medical Faculty, Eskisehir Osmangazi University, Turkey

5 Neurology Department, Istanbul Bagcilar Education and Research Hospital, Turkey

6 Neurology Department, Medical Faculty, Marmara University, Turkey

7 Neurology Department, Acibadem Eskisehir Hospital, Turkey

*Address all correspondence to: demetozbabalik@gmail.com

References

[1] Derouesné C. Alzheimer and Alzheimer's disease: The present enlighted by the past. An historical approach. Psychologie & Neuropsychiatrie du Vieillissement. 2008;**6**(2):115-128

[2] Hardy JA, Higgins GA. Alzheimer's disease: The amyloid cascade hypothesis. Science. 1992;**256**(5054):184

[3] Herrup K. The case for rejecting the amyloid cascade hypothesis. Nature Neuroscience. 2015;**18**(6):794

[4] Iqbal K, Liu F, Gong C-X, Alonso AC, Grundke-Iqbal I. Mechanisms of tau-induced neurodegeneration. Acta Neuropathologica. 2009;**118**(1):53-69

[5] Alonso AC, Zaidi T, Grundke-Iqbal I, Iqbal K. Role of abnormally phosphorylated tau in the breakdown of microtubules in Alzheimer disease. Proceedings of the National Academy of Sciences. 1994;**91**(12):5562-5566

[6] Beal MF. Oxidatively modified proteins in aging and disease1, 2. Free Radical Biology and Medicine. 2002;**32**(9):797-803

[7] Gemma C, Vila J, Bachstetter A, Bickford PC. Oxidative Stress and the Aging Brain: From Theory to Prevention. 2007

[8] Janelsins MC, Mastrangelo MA, Oddo S, LaFerla FM, Federoff HJ, Bowers WJ. Early correlation of microglial activation with enhanced tumor necrosis factor-alpha and monocyte chemoattractant protein-1 expression specifically within the entorhinal cortex of triple transgenic Alzheimer's disease mice. Journal of Neuroinflammation. 2005;**2**(1):23

[9] Bellucci A, Westwood AJ, Ingram E, Casamenti F, Goedert M, Spillantini MG. Induction of inflammatory mediators and microglial activation in mice transgenic for mutant human P301S tau protein. The American Journal of Pathology. 2004;**165**(5):1643-1652

[10] Sastre M, Dewachter I, Landreth GE, Willson TM, Klockgether T, Van Leuven F, et al. Nonsteroidal anti-inflammatory drugs and peroxisome proliferator-activated receptor-γ agonists modulate immunostimulated processing of amyloid precursor protein through regulation of β-secretase. Journal of Neuroscience. 2003;**23**(30):9796-9804

[11] Szekely CA, Breitner JC, Fitzpatrick AL, Rea TD, Psaty BM, Kuller LH, et al. NSAID use and dementia risk in the cardiovascular health study: Role of APOE and NSAID type. Neurology. 2008;**70**(1):17-24

[12] Smith DG, Cappai R, Barnham KJ. The redox chemistry of the Alzheimer's disease amyloid β peptide. Biochimica et Biophysica Acta (BBA)—Biomembranes. 2007;**1768**(8):1976-1990

[13] Swerdlow RH, Khan SM. A "mitochondrial cascade hypothesis" for sporadic Alzheimer's disease. Medical Hypotheses. 2004;**63**(1):8-20

[14] Rivera EJ, Goldin A, Fulmer N, Tavares R, Wands JR, de la Monte SM. Insulin and insulin-like growth factor expression and function deteriorate with progression of Alzheimer's disease: Link to brain reductions in acetylcholine. Journal of Alzheimer's Disease. 2005;**8**(3):247-268

[15] Qaseem A, Snow V, Cross JT, Forciea MA, Hopkins R, Shekelle P, et al. Current pharmacologic treatment of dementia: A clinical practice guideline from the American College of Physicians and the American Academy of Family Physicians. Annals of Internal Medicine. 2008;**148**(5):370-378

[16] Norton S, Matthews FE, Barnes DE, Yaffe K, Brayne C. Potential for primary prevention of Alzheimer's disease: An analysis of population-based data. The Lancet Neurology. 2014;**13**(8):788-794

[17] Barage SH, Sonawane KD. Amyloid cascade hypothesis: Pathogenesis and therapeutic strategies in Alzheimer's disease. Neuropeptides. 2015;**52**:1-18

[18] Tayeb HO, Yang HD, Price BH, Tarazi FI. Pharmacotherapies for Alzheimer's disease: Beyond cholinesterase inhibitors. Pharmacology & Therapeutics. 2012;**134**(1):8-25

[19] Pedersen JT, Sigurdsson EM. Tau immunotherapy for Alzheimer's disease. Trends in Molecular Medicine. 2015;**21**(6):394-402

[20] Cummings JL, Morstorf T, Zhong K. Alzheimer's disease drug-development pipeline: Few candidates, frequent failures. Alzheimer's Research & Therapy. 2014;**6**(4):37

[21] Becker RE, Greig NH, Giacobini E. Why do so many drugs for Alzheimer's disease fail in development? Time for new methods and new practices. Journal of Alzheimer's Disease. 2008;**15**(2):303-325

[22] Anand A, Patience AA, Sharma N, Khurana N. The present and future of pharmacotherapy of Alzheimer's disease: A comprehensive review. European Journal of Pharmacology. 2017;**815**:364-375

[23] Racchi M, Mazzucchelli M, Porrello E, Lanni C, Govoni S. Acetylcholinesterase inhibitors: Novel activities of old molecules. Pharmacological Research. 2004;**50**(4):441-451

[24] Arrieta L, López-Arrieta JM, Schneider L. Metrifonate for Alzheimer's disease. Cochrane Database of Systematic Reviews. 2006;(2)

[25] Higgins JP, Flicker L. Lecithin for dementia and cognitive impairment. Cochrane Database of Systematic Reviews. 2000:4

[26] Tabet N, Feldman H. Ibuprofen for Alzheimer's disease. Cochrane Database of Systematic Reviews. 2003;(2)

[27] Reines S, Block G, Morris J, Liu G, Nessly M, Lines C, et al. Rofecoxib: No effect on Alzheimer's disease in a 1-year, randomized, blinded, controlled study. Neurology. 2004;**62**(1):66-71

[28] Jaturapatporn D, Isaac MGEKN, McCleery J, Tabet N. Aspirin, steroidal and non-steroidal anti-inflammatory drugs for the treatment of Alzheimer's disease. Cochrane Database of Systematic Reviews. 2012;(2)

[29] Chau S, Herrmann N, Ruthirakuhan MT, Chen JJ, Lanctot KL. Latrepirdine for Alzheimer's disease. The Cochrane Library. 2015

[30] Birks J, Flicker L. Selegiline for Alzheimer's disease. Cochrane Database of Systematic Reviews. 2003;(1)

[31] Shepherd J. A prospective study of Pravastatin in the Elderly at Risk (PROSPER). Lancet. 2002;**360**:685-696

[32] McGuinness B, Craig D, Bullock R, Passmore P. Statins for the prevention of dementia. The Cochrane Library. 2016

[33] Burckhardt M, Herke M, Wustmann T, Watzke S, Langer G, Fink A. Omega-3 fatty acids for the treatment of dementia. The Cochrane Library. 2016

[34] Kryscio RJ, Abner EL, Caban-Holt A, Lovell M, Goodman P, Darke AK, et al. Association of antioxidant supplement use and dementia in the prevention of Alzheimer's disease by vitamin E and selenium trial (PREADViSE). JAMA Neurology. 2017;**74**(5):567-573

[35] Farina N, Isaac MGEKN, Clark AR, Rusted J, Tabet N. Vitamin E

for Alzheimer's dementia and mild cognitive impairment. Cochrane Database of Dystematic Reviews. 2012;**2012**(11):CD002854

[36] Li M-M, Yu J-T, Wang H-F, Jiang T, Wang J, Meng X-F, et al. Efficacy of vitamins B supplementation on mild cognitive impairment and Alzheimer's disease: A systematic review and meta-analysis. Current Alzheimer Research. 2014;**11**(9):844-852

[37] Hudson SA, Tabet N. Acetyl-l-carnitine for dementia. Cochrane Database of Systematic Reviews. 2003;(2)

[38] Flicker L, Evans JG. Piracetam for dementia or cognitive impairment. Cochrane Database of Systematic Reviews. 2004;(1)

[39] Doody RS, Raman R, Farlow M, Iwatsubo T, Vellas B, Joffe S, et al. A phase 3 trial of semagacestat for treatment of Alzheimer's disease. New England Journal of Medicine. 2013;**369**(4):341-350

[40] Green RC, Schneider LS, Amato DA, Beelen AP, Wilcock G, Swabb EA, et al. Effect of tarenflurbil on cognitive decline and activities of daily living in patients with mild Alzheimer disease: A randomized controlled trial. Journal of the American Medical Association. 2009;**302**(23):2557-2564

[41] Abushouk AI, Elmaraezy A, Aglan A, Salama R, Fouda S, Fouda R, et al. Bapineuzumab for mild to moderate Alzheimer's disease: A meta-analysis of randomized controlled trials. BMC Neurology. 2017;**17**(1):66

[42] Honig LS, Vellas B, Woodward M, Boada M, Bullock R, Borrie M, et al. Trial of solanezumab for mild dementia due to Alzheimer's disease. New England Journal of Medicine. 2018;**378**(4):321-330

[43] LaFerla FM, Green KN, Oddo S. Intracellular amyloid-β in Alzheimer's disease. Nature Reviews Neuroscience. 2007;**8**(7):499

[44] Do TD, LaPointe NE, Nelson R, Krotee P, Hayden EY, Ulrich B, et al. Amyloid β-protein C-terminal fragments: Formation of cylindrins and β-barrels. Journal of the American Chemical Society. 2016;**138**(2):549-557

[45] Bode DC, Baker MD, Viles JH. Ion channel formation by amyloid-β42 oligomers but not amyloid-β40 in cellular membranes. Journal of Biological Chemistry. 2017;**292**(4):1404-1413

[46] van Dyck CH. Anti-amyloid-β monoclonal antibodies for Alzheimer's disease: Pitfalls and promise. Biological Psychiatry. 2018;**83**(4):311-319

[47] Tsang JY, Lee MA, Chan T-H, Li J, Ni Y-B, Shao Y, et al. Proteolytic cleavage of amyloid precursor protein by ADAM10 mediates proliferation and migration in breast cancer. eBioMedicine. 2018;**38**:89-99

[48] Kumar D, Ganeshpurkar A, Kumar D, Modi GP, Gupta SK, Singh SK. Secretase inhibitors for the treatment of Alzheimer's disease: Long road ahead. European Journal of Medicinal Chemistry. 2018

[49] Hung S-Y, Fu W-M. Drug candidates in clinical trials for Alzheimer's disease. Journal of Biomedical Science. 2017;**24**(1):47

[50] Gilman S, Koller M, Black R, Jenkins L, Griffith S, Fox N, et al. Clinical effects of Aβ immunization (AN1792) in patients with AD in AN interrupted trial. Neurology. 2005;**64**(9):1553-1562

[51] Montoliu-Gaya L, Villegas S. Aβ-immunotherapeutic strategies: A wide range of approaches for Alzheimer's disease treatment. Expert Reviews in Molecular Medicine. 2016;**18**

[52] Sarazin M, Dorothée G, de Souza LC, Aucouturier P. Immunotherapy in Alzheimer's disease: Do we have all the pieces of the puzzle? Biological Psychiatry. 2013;**74**(5):329-332

[53] Adolfsson O, Pihlgren M, Toni N, Varisco Y, Buccarello AL, Antoniello K, et al. An effector-reduced anti-β-amyloid (Aβ) antibody with unique aβ binding properties promotes neuroprotection and glial engulfment of Aβ. Journal of Neuroscience. 2012;**32**(28):9677-9689

[54] Ultsch M, Li B, Maurer T, Mathieu M, Adolfsson O, Muhs A, et al. Structure of crenezumab complex with Aβ shows loss of β-hairpin. Scientific Reports. 2016;**6**:39374

[55] Bateman RJ, Benzinger TL, Berry S, Clifford DB, Duggan C, Fagan AM, et al. The DIAN-TU next generation Alzheimer's prevention trial: Adaptive design and disease progression model. Alzheimer's & Dementia. 2017;**13**(1):8-19

[56] Lasser R, Ostrowitzki S, Scheltens P, Boada M, Dubois B, Dorflinger E, et al. Efficacy and safety of gantenerumab in prodromal Alzheimer's disease: Results from scarlet road—A global, multicenter trial. Alzheimer's & Dementia: The Journal of the Alzheimer's Association. 2015;**11**(7):P331-P3P2

[57] Sevigny J, Chiao P, Bussière T, Weinreb PH, Williams L, Maier M, et al. The antibody aducanumab reduces Aβ plaques in Alzheimer's disease. Nature. 2016;**537**(7618):50-56

[58] Siemers ER, Sundell KL, Carlson C, Case M, Sethuraman G, Liu-Seifert H, et al. Phase 3 solanezumab trials: Secondary outcomes in mild Alzheimer's disease patients. Alzheimer's & Dementia. 2016;**12**(2):110-120

[59] Schenk D, Barbour R, Dunn W, Gordon G, Grajeda H, Guido T, et al. Immunization with amyloid-β attenuates Alzheimer-disease-like pathology in the PDAPP mouse. Nature. 1999;**400**(6740):173

[60] Panza F, Solfrizzi V, Imbimbo BP, Tortelli R, Santamato A, Logroscino G. Amyloid-based immunotherapy for Alzheimer's disease in the time of prevention trials: The way forward. Expert Review of Clinical Immunology. 2014;**10**(3):405-419

[61] Davtyan H, Bacon A, Petrushina I, Zagorski K, Cribbs DH, Ghochikyan A, et al. Immunogenicity of DNA-and recombinant protein-based Alzheimer disease epitope vaccines. Human Vaccines & Immunotherapeutics. 2014;**10**(5):1248-1255

[62] Sperling RA, Rentz DM, Johnson KA, Karlawish J, Donohue M, Salmon DP, et al. The A4 study: Stopping AD before symptoms begin? Science Translational Medicine. 2014;**6**(228):228fs13-fs13

[63] Terwel D, Dewachter I, Van Leuven F. Axonal transport, tau protein, and neurodegeneration in Alzheimer's disease. Neuromolecular Medicine. 2002;**2**(2):151-165

[64] Medina M, Hernández F, Avila J. New features about tau function and dysfunction. Biomolecules. 2016;**6**(2):21

[65] Sontag J-M, Sontag E. Protein phosphatase 2A dysfunction in Alzheimer's disease. Frontiers in Molecular Neuroscience. 2014;**7**(2):21

[66] Bruch J, Xu H, Rösler TW, De Andrade A, Kuhn PH, Lichtenthaler SF, et al. PERK activation mitigates tau pathology in vitro and in vivo. EMBO Molecular Medicine. 2017;**9**(3):371-384

[67] Wischik CM, Staff RT, Wischik DJ, Bentham P, Murray AD, Storey J, et al. Tau aggregation inhibitor therapy: An exploratory phase 2 study

in mild or moderate Alzheimer's disease. Journal of Alzheimer's Disease. 2015;**44**(2):705-720

[68] Gauthier S, Feldman HH, Schneider LS, Wilcock GK, Frisoni GB, Hardlund JH, et al. Efficacy and safety of tau-aggregation inhibitor therapy in patients with mild or moderate Alzheimer's disease: A randomised, controlled, double-blind, parallel-arm, phase 3 trial. The Lancet. 2016;**388**(10062):2873-2884

[69] Guo T, Noble W, Hanger DP. Roles of tau protein in health and disease. Acta Neuropathologica. 2017;**133**(5):665-704

[70] Hu W, Zhang X, Tung YC, Xie S, Liu F, Iqbal K. Hyperphosphorylation determines both the spread and the morphology of tau pathology. Alzheimer's & Dementia. 2016;**12**(10):1066-1077

[71] Alonso AC, Grundke-Iqbal I, Iqbal K. Alzheimer's disease hyperphosphorylated tau sequesters normal tau into tangles of filaments and disassembles microtubules. Nature Medicine. 1996;**2**(7):783-787

[72] Theunis C, Crespo-Biel N, Gafner V, Pihlgren M, López-Deber MP, Reis P, et al. Efficacy and safety of a liposome-based vaccine against protein tau, assessed in tau. P301L mice that model tauopathy. PLoS One. 2013;**8**(8):e72301

[73] Lünemann JD, Nimmerjahn F, Dalakas MC. Intravenous immunoglobulin in neurology—Mode of action and clinical efficacy. Nature Reviews Neurology. 2015;**11**(2):80

[74] Relkin NR, Thomas RG, Rissman RA, Brewer JB, Rafii MS, Van Dyck CH, et al. A phase 3 trial of IV immunoglobulin for Alzheimer disease. Neurology. 2017. DOI: 10.1212/WNL.0000000000003904

[75] Min S-W, Chen X, Tracy TE, Li Y, Zhou Y, Wang C, et al. Critical role of acetylation in tau-mediated neurodegeneration and cognitive deficits. Nature Medicine. 2015;**21**(10):1154

[76] Ursan ID, Jiang R, Pickard EM, Lee TA, Ng D, Pickard AS. Emergence of BCR-ABL kinase domain mutations associated with newly diagnosed chronic myeloid leukemia: A meta-analysis of clinical trials of tyrosine kinase inhibitors. Journal of Managed Care & Specialty Pharmacy. 2015;**21**(2):114-122

[77] Medina M. An overview on the clinical development of tau-based therapeutics. International Journal of Molecular Sciences. 2018;**19**(4):1160

[78] Barrera-Ocampo A, Lopera F. Amyloid-beta immunotherapy: The hope for Alzheimer disease. Colombia Médica. 2016;**47**(4):203-212

[79] Wang S-J, Wang K-Y, Wang W-C. Mechanisms underlying the riluzole inhibition of glutamate release from rat cerebral cortex nerve terminals (synaptosomes). Neuroscience. 2004;**125**(1):191-201

[80] Fumagalli E, Funicello M, Rauen T, Gobbi M, Mennini T. Riluzole enhances the activity of glutamate transporters GLAST, GLT1 and EAAC1. European Journal of Pharmacology. 2008;**578**(2-3):171-176

[81] Grant P, Song JY, Swedo SE. Review of the use of the glutamate antagonist riluzole in psychiatric disorders and a description of recent use in childhood obsessive-compulsive disorder. Journal of Child and Adolescent Psychopharmacology. 2010;**20**(4):309-315

[82] Hunsberger HC, Weitzner DS, Rudy CC, Hickman JE, Libell EM, Speer RR, et al. Riluzole rescues glutamate alterations, cognitive deficits, and tau pathology associated with P301L tau

expression. Journal of Neurochemistry. 2015;**135**(2):381-394

[83] Knowles JK, Simmons DA, Nguyen T-VV, Vander Griend L, Xie Y, Zhang H, et al. A small molecule p75NTR ligand prevents cognitive deficits and neurite degeneration in an Alzheimer's mouse model. Neurobiology of Aging. 2013;**34**(8):2052-2063

[84] Nguyen T-VV, Shen L, Vander Griend L, Quach LN, Belichenko NP, Saw N, et al. Small molecule p75 NTR ligands reduce pathological phosphorylation and misfolding of tau, inflammatory changes, cholinergic degeneration, and cognitive deficits in AβPP L/S transgenic mice. Journal of Alzheimer's Disease. 2014;**42**(2):459-483

[85] Cao J, Hou J, Ping J, Cai D. Advances in developing novel therapeutic strategies for Alzheimer's disease. Molecular Neurodegeneration. 2018;**13**(1):64

[86] Eimer WA, Kumar V, Kumar D, Shanmugam NKN, Washicosky KJ, Rodriguez AS, et al. Alzheimer's disease-associated β-amyloid is rapidly seeded by herpesviridae to protect against brain infection. 2018

[87] Kumar DKV, Choi SH, Washicosky KJ, Eimer WA, Tucker S, Ghofrani J, et al. Amyloid-β peptide protects against microbial infection in mouse and worm models of Alzheimer's disease. Science Translational Medicine. 2016;**8**(340):340ra72-340ra72

[88] Craft S, Baker LD, Montine TJ, Minoshima S, Watson GS, Claxton A, et al. Intranasal insulin therapy for Alzheimer disease and amnestic mild cognitive impairment: A pilot clinical trial. Archives of Neurology. 2012;**69**(1):29-38

[89] Reger MA, Watson G, Green PS, Baker LD, Cholerton B, Fishel MA, et al. Intranasal insulin administration dose-dependently modulates verbal memory and plasma amyloid-β in memory-impaired older adults. Journal of Alzheimer's Disease. 2008;**13**(3):323-331

[90] Morris MC, Tangney CC, Wang Y, Sacks FM, Barnes LL, Bennett DA, et al. MIND diet slows cognitive decline with aging. Alzheimer's & Dementia. 2015;**11**(9):1015-1022

[91] Morris MC, Tangney CC, Wang Y, Sacks FM, Bennett DA, Aggarwal NT. MIND diet associated with reduced incidence of Alzheimer's disease. Alzheimer's & Dementia. 2015;**11**(9):1007-1014

[92] Reger M, Watson G, Green P, Wilkinson C, Baker L, Cholerton B, et al. Intranasal insulin improves cognition and modulates β-amyloid in early AD. Neurology. 2008;**70**(6):440-448

[93] Association As. 2016 Alzheimer's disease facts and figures. Alzheimer's & Dementia. 2016;**12**(4):459-509

[94] Zou Z, Liu C, Che C, Huang H. Clinical genetics of Alzheimer's disease. BioMed Research International. 2014;**2014**

[95] Zhong N, Weisgraber KH. Understanding the association of apolipoprotein E4 with Alzheimer disease: Clues from its structure. Journal of Biological Chemistry. 2009;**284**(10):6027-6031

[96] Karch CM, Goate AM. Alzheimer's disease risk genes and mechanisms of disease pathogenesis. Biological Psychiatry. 2015;**77**(1):43-51

[97] Y-w Z, Thompson R, Zhang H, Xu H. APP processing in Alzheimer's disease. Molecular Brain. 2011;**4**(1):3

[98] Larner A. Presenilin-1 mutations in Alzheimer's disease: An update on

genotype-phenotype relationships. Journal of Alzheimer's Disease. 2013;**37**(4):653-659

[99] Bekris LM, Yu C-E, Bird TD, Tsuang DW. Genetics of Alzheimer disease. Journal of Geriatric Psychiatry and Neurology. 2010;**23**(4):213-227

[100] Jayadev S, Leverenz JB, Steinbart E, Stahl J, Klunk W, Yu C-E, et al. Alzheimer's disease phenotypes and genotypes associated with mutations in presenilin 2. Brain. 2010;**133**(4):1143-1154

[101] Marioni RE, Harris SE, Zhang Q, McRae AF, Hagenaars SP, Hill WD, et al. GWAS on family history of Alzheimer's disease. Translational Psychiatry. 2018;**8**(1):99

[102] Carty NC, Nash K, Lee D, Mercer M, Gottschall PE, Meyers C, et al. Adeno-associated viral (AAV) serotype 5 vector mediated gene delivery of endothelin-converting enzyme reduces Aβ deposits in APP+ PS1 transgenic mice. Molecular Therapy. 2008;**16**(9):1580-1586

[103] Shimada M, Abe S, Takahashi T, Shiozaki K, Okuda M, Mizukami H, et al. Prophylaxis and treatment of Alzheimer's disease by delivery of an adeno-associated virus encoding a monoclonal antibody targeting the amyloid Beta protein. PLoS One. 2013;**8**(3):e57606

[104] Martinez-Morales P, Revilla A, Ocana I, Gonzalez C, Sainz P, McGuire D, et al. Progress in stem cell therapy for major human neurological disorders. Stem Cell Reviews and Reports. 2013;**9**(5):685-699

[105] Lunn JS, Sakowski SA, Hur J, Feldman EL. Stem cell technology for neurodegenerative diseases. Annals of Neurology. 2011;**70**(3):353-361

[106] Tang J, Xu H, Fan X, Li D, Rancourt D, Zhou G, et al. Embryonic stem cell-derived neural precursor cells improve memory dysfunction in Aβ (1-40) injured rats. Neuroscience Research. 2008;**62**(2):86-96

[107] Kwak K-A, Lee S-P, Yang J-Y, Park Y-S. Current perspectives regarding stem cell-based therapy for Alzheimer's disease. Stem Cells International. 2018;**2018**

[108] Jin X, Lin T, Xu Y. Stem cell therapy and immunological rejection in animal models. Current Molecular Pharmacology. 2016;**9**(4):284-288

[109] Araki R, Uda M, Hoki Y, Sunayama M, Nakamura M, Ando S, et al. Negligible immunogenicity of terminally differentiated cells derived from induced pluripotent or embryonic stem cells. Nature. 2013;**494**(7435):100

[110] Lee JH, Oh I-H, Lim HK. Stem cell therapy: A prospective treatment for Alzheimer's disease. Psychiatry Investigation. 2016;**13**(6):583-589

[111] Takahashi K, Tanabe K, Ohnuki M, Narita M, Ichisaka T, Tomoda K, et al. Induction of pluripotent stem cells from adult human fibroblasts by defined factors. Cell. 2007;**131**(5):861-872

[112] Fang Y, Gao T, Zhang B, Pu J. Recent advances: Decoding Alzheimer's disease with stem cells. Frontiers in Aging Neuroscience. 2018;**10**:77

[113] Yang J, Li S, He X-B, Cheng C, Le W. Induced pluripotent stem cells in Alzheimer's disease: Applications for disease modeling and cell-replacement therapy. Molecular Neurodegeneration. 2016;**11**(1):39

[114] Yagi T, Ito D, Okada Y, Akamatsu W, Nihei Y, Yoshizaki T, et al. Modeling familial Alzheimer's disease with induced pluripotent stem cells. Human Molecular Genetics. 2011;**20**(23):4530-4539

[115] Takamatsu K, Ikeda T, Haruta M, Matsumura K, Ogi Y, Nakagata N, et al. Degradation of amyloid beta by human induced pluripotent stem cell-derived macrophages expressing Neprilysin-2. Stem Cell Research. 2014;**13**(3):442-453

[116] Lister R, Pelizzola M, Kida YS, Hawkins RD, Nery JR, Hon G, et al. Hotspots of aberrant epigenomic reprogramming in human induced pluripotent stem cells. Nature. 2011;**471**(7336):68

[117] Park D, Yang G, Bae DK, Lee SH, Yang YH, Kyung J, et al. Human adipose tissue-derived mesenchymal stem cells improve cognitive function and physical activity in ageing mice. Journal of Neuroscience Research. 2013;**91**(5):660-670

[118] Zilka N, Zilkova M, Kazmerova Z, Sarissky M, Cigankova V, Novak M. Mesenchymal stem cells rescue the Alzheimer's disease cell model from cell death induced by misfolded truncated tau. Neuroscience. 2011;**193**:330-337

[119] Yang H, Xie ZH, Wei LF, Yang HN, Yang SN, Zhu ZY, et al. Human umbilical cord mesenchymal stem cell-derived neuron-like cells rescue memory deficits and reduce amyloid-beta deposition in an AβPP/PS1 transgenic mouse model. Stem Cell Research & Therapy. 2013;**4**(4):76

[120] J-s B, Jin HK, Lee JK, Richardson JC, Carter JE. Bone marrow-derived mesenchymal stem cells contribute to the reduction of amyloid-β deposits and the improvement of synaptic transmission in a mouse model of pre-dementia Alzheimer's disease. Current Alzheimer Research. 2013;**10**(5):524-531

[121] Duncan T, Valenzuela M. Alzheimer's disease, dementia, and stem cell therapy. Stem Cell Research & Therapy. 2017;**8**(1):111

[122] Park D, Yang Y-H, Bae DK, Lee SH, Yang G, Kyung J, et al. Improvement of cognitive function and physical activity of aging mice by human neural stem cells over-expressing choline acetyltransferase. Neurobiology of Aging. 2013;**34**(11):2639-2646

Section 3

Newer Developments in Geriatrics

Chapter 7

Genetics and Acquired Hearing Loss

Moza Al-Kowari and Meritxell Espino-Guarch

Abstract

Hearing loss (HL) is a worldwide disease with substantial economic costs for the public health. Around 466 million people have disabling hearing loss and the WHO estimated that by 2050 over 900 million people will suffer hearing loss. Several factors including infections, noise-exposure, ototoxic medications or genetic disorders could cause hearing impairment. Hearing devices such as cochlear implants and aids are the current therapies. Although the prevalence of hearing loss is very high, alternative treatments as pharmaceutical agents are currently insufficient. Within the past years, increased knowledge on hearing loss etiology and physiopathology opened new opportunities for future research towards hearing loss treatment. Here we aim to review current bibliography on genetics factors involved in hearing loss.

Keywords: hearing loss, genetics, syndromic, non-syndromic, age-related

1. Introduction

The World Health Organization (WHO) defines hearing loss (HL) as the inability to perceive the sounds with different grades of impairment, from slight to profound including deafness [1].

Sound waves move from outer (or external) to middle and then to the inner ear, three anatomically distinct structures of the ear which transmit the sound to a signal into the brain. The sound waves travel down the cannel of the outer and middle ear until hitting the tympanic membrane. Vibrations from the middle ear create movement of the fluid in the inner ear. This movement of the fluid is transmitted through the tectorial membrane to the hair cells in the organ of Corti, then the stimulus is transmitted by electric signals up to the auditory nerve to the brain. The brain interprets the electrical signals as sound. **Figure 1** shows the different compartment of the ear as described above.

Depending on the compartment affected, hearing loss could be classified as *conductive* or *sensorineural*. Conductive hearing loss is when the outer and middle ear are affected, and it results in the inability to transmit sound waves to the inner ear [3]. On the other hand, impairments in the inner ear are known as sensorineural [4]. Conductive hearing loss could be treated by medication, surgery cochlear implants or hearing aids, meanwhile sensorineural is mostly irreversible because of the complexity of the structure, the limited regeneration and access to the sensory structures in the cochlea [5].

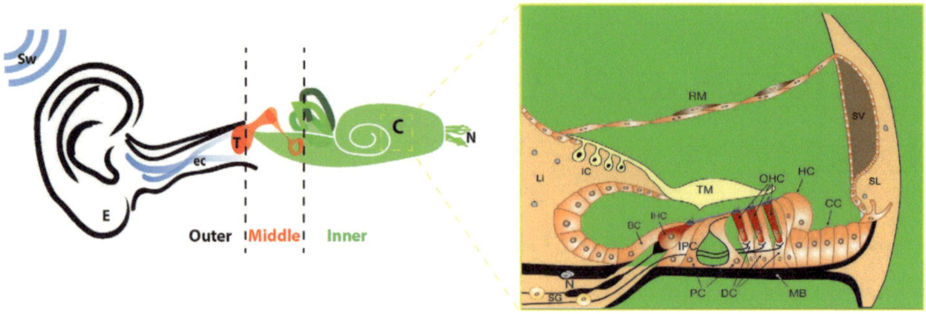

Figure 1.
Scheme of hearing system from external ear to inner ear. Path of the sound waves (in blue) through outer, middle and inner ear is represented where Sw, sound waves; E, external ear; ec, ear canal; T, tympanic membrane; C, cochlea; N, auditory nerve. Magnification of the cochlea structures (adapted from Sanchez-Calderon et al. [2]) is shown framed in yellow where BC, border cells; CC, Claudius's cells; DC, Deiter's cells; HC, Hensen's cells; IC, intermediate cells; IHC, inner hair cells; IPC, inner phalangeal cells; Li, spiral limbus; N, cochlear neurons; MB, Basilar Membrane; OHC, outer hair cells; PC, pillar cells; RM, Reisner's membrane; SG, spiral ganglion; SL, spiral ligament; SV, stria vascularis and TM, tectorial membrane.

2. Hearing loss etiology

There are several causes of hearing loss affecting over 500 million people worldwide [6]. Approximately 50% of the hearing impairment has a genetic etiology, the remaining cases are attributed to external factor such as noise or injury (acquired/spontaneous). In addition, the contribution of both (genetic predisposition and environment) is very common as found in age-related hearing loss [7, 8].

Inherited hearing loss can be autosomal recessive or dominant, X-linked or mitochondrial-related. The autosomal recessive hearing loss is caused by pathogenic variant in both alleles (the child inherits them from both parents). Autosomal dominant inheritance occurs when variants in one single allele are able to cause hearing loss. Independent of the inheritance pattern, genetics of hearing loss are classified as syndromic when they are associated with pathologies in other organs or malformations of the external ear and non-syndromic [6]. Approximately 30% of hearing loss are syndromic whereas the 70% remaining are non-syndromic [9]. Each type of hearing loss (syndromic and non-syndromic) is further classified according to the mode of inheritance into autosomal recessive, autosomal dominant, X-linked and mitochondrial hearing loss.

2.1 Syndromic hearing loss

Syndromic hearing loss (SHL) is a form of hearing impairments in which it is associated with other diseases or symptoms. Most commonly SHL is associated with diseases that affect eyes, nervous system and skin. SHL accounts for 30% of hereditary hearing loss and can be inherited in an autosomal recessive, dominant and X-linked patterns. Moreover, several genes described in SHL are also causing non-syndromic hearing loss (NSHL) such as mutations in CDH23 gene causing either Usher syndrome type 1D and autosomal recessive NSHL (DFNB12) (OMIM: 605516) [10].

2.1.1 Autosomal dominant SHL

Waardenburg syndrome (WS) is first described in 1951 by Waardenburg. It is one of the most common congenital, sensorineural SHL [11]. Clinical symptoms include lateral displacement of the inner canthus of the eye (dystopia canthorum), pigmentations of the hair, eye and skin. It is estimated that WS is accounting for 2–5% of congenital hearing loss cases. According to the presence or absence of the clinical symptoms, Waardenburg syndrome is divided into four subtypes: WS1, WS2, WS3 and WS4. Patients with WS1, usually has dystopia canthorum, while patient with WS2 are not. WS3 also called Klein-Waardenburg syndrome characterized by dystopia canthorum and upper limb abnormalities. The last type WS4 also called Waardenburg-Shah syndrome is associated with Hirschsprung disease. Patients with WS4 are suffering from blockage of the large intestine and neurological defects. According to the hereditary hearing loss homepage, six genes are associated with WS (**Table 1**) [12]. These genes are essential for the development of melanocytes and have a major role in the function of the inner ear.

Branchio-Oto-Renal Syndrome (BOR) is the second common autosomal dominant congenital SHL. It is characterized by malformations in the ears and is associated with different types of hearing loss: conductive, sensorineural and mixed hearing loss. Moreover, BOR syndrome is affecting kidneys structure and functions which results in renal abnormalities [13]. The frequency of BOR syndrome is estimated to be 1 in 40,000 individuals. Mutations in Eyes Absent homolog 1 (*EYA1*), Sine Oculis Homebox 5 (*SIX5*) and Sine Oculis Homebox 1 (*SIX1*) genes are found to be associated with BOR syndrome (**Table 1**). These genes are required for normal embryonic development of different organs including both the kidneys and the ears.

Syndrome	Gene	OMIM entry	Inheritance
Alport syndrome	*COL4A3*	120070	AR
	COL4A4	120131	AR
	COL4A5	303630	XL
Branchio-Oto-Renal syndrome	*EYA1*	601653	AD
	SIX5	600963	AD
	SIX1	601205	AD
CHARGE syndrome	*CHD7*	608892	AD
	SEMA3E	608166	AD
Jervell and Lange-Nielsen syndrome	*KNCQ1*	607542	AR
	KCNE1	176261	AR
Norrie disease	*NDP*	300658	XL
Pendred syndrome	*SLC26A4*	605646	AR
	KCNJ10	602208	AR
	FOX11	601093	AR
Perrault syndrome	*HSD17B4*	601860	AR
	HARS2	600783	AR
	CLPP	601119	AR
	LARS2	604544	AR
	TWNK	606075	AR
	ERAL1	607435	AR
Stickler syndrome	*COL2A1*	120140	AD
	COL11A1	120280	AD
	COL11A2	120290	AD
	COL9A1	120210	AR
	COL9A2	120260	AR

Syndrome	Gene	OMIM entry	Inheritance
Treacher Collins syndrome	*TCOF1*	606847	AD
	POLR1D	613715	AD
	POLR1C	610060	AD
Usher syndrome	*MYO7A*	276903	AD
	USH1C	605242	AR
	CDH23	605516	AR
	PCDH15	605514	AR
	SANS	607696	AR
	USH2A	608400	AR
	ADGRV1	602851	AR
	WHRN	607928	AR
	CLRN1	606397	AR
	HARS	142810	AR
Waardenburg syndrome	*PAX3*	606597	AD
	MITF	156845	AD
	SNAI2	602150	AD
	SOX10	602229	AD
	PAX3	606597	AD
	EDNRB	131244	AR
	EDN3	131242	AR
	SOX10	602229	AR

Table 1.
List of syndromic hearing loss and its associated genes [12].

CHARGE syndrome is another form of autosomal dominant hearing loss syndrome that affects several organs. Patients with CHARGE syndrome are characterized by different phenotypes, from which the name of the syndrome comes from, this includes: Coloboma, Heart defects, Atresia choanae, growth Retardation, Genital abnormalities and Ear abnormalities. The degree of abnormalities varies from one patient to another. It ranges from very severe and vital cases to minor phenotypes. The prevalence of CHARGE syndrome estimated to be 1 in 8500 to 10,000 newborns worldwide. Chromodomain helicase DNA-binding protein-7 (*CHD7*) is found to be the common cause of CHARGE syndrome. *CHD7* is a transcription factor protein that regulates chromatin [14].

2.1.2 Autosomal recessive SHL

Usher syndrome is an autosomal recessive sensorineural hearing loss (SNHL) with retinitis [15]. According to the clinical phenotype, Usher syndrome is classified to three main types: Usher 1 (USH1), Usher 2 (USH2) and Usher 3 (USH3). USH1 is characterized by severe to profound SNHL, severe vestibular impairments and early onset retinitis pigmentosa. Mutations in several genes are found to be the cause of USH1 syndrome (**Table 1**). The most common genes causing USH1 are *MYO7A* and *CHD23*. Both genes are important for the development and function of inner ear hair cells. Patients with USH2 are found to suffer from moderate to severe SNHL with mid onset retinitis pigmentosa and no vestibular impairment. Usherin (*USH2A*) and Adhesion-G protein coupled receptor VI (*ADGRVI*) are found to be mutated in patients diagnosed with USH2. The last type is USH3 that is characterized by variable phenotypes of progressive hearing loss, vestibular impairment and late onset retinitis pigmentosa. The prevalence of Usher syndrome is estimated to be 1 in 6000 to 10,000 with USH1 and USH2 being the most common types.

The second common autosomal recessive SHL is *Pendred Syndrome* which is characterized by hearing loss and thyroid enlargement [16]. The hearing loss ranges from severe to profound are usually developed at early childhood [17]. A characteristic feature of Pendred syndrome is the Mondini malformation which is a combination of enlarged vestibular aqueduct and abnormal shape of the cochlea. The prevalence of Pendred syndrome is ranged from 1 to 7.5 per 100,000 newborns. Three genes are found to be mutated in patients with Pendred syndrome: *SLC26A4* which encodes for sodium-independent transporter of chloride iodide protein called Pendrin [18], *FOXI1* [19] and *KCNJ10* [20]. Approximately 50% of Pendred syndrome patients had mutations in *SLC26A4* gene, whereas the other two genes mutated in Pendred syndrome patients account for less than 2% of the cases are).

Jervell and Lange-Nielsen Syndrome is the third common autosomal recessive syndromic hearing loss. This condition is characterized by profound hearing loss with arrhythmia and long QT interval in the electrocardiogram that may result in heart failure and sudden death [21]. The prevalence of this syndrome is estimated to affect 1.6–6 per million people worldwide [22]. Genes found to be mutated in patients with this syndrome are potassium channel voltage-gated KQT-like subfamily member 1 (*KCNQ1*) [23] and potassium channel voltage-gated ISK-related subfamily member 1 (*KCNE1*) [24] with majority of the mutations (90%) occurs in *KCNQ1*. These channels are important for the movement of the potassium ions in order to maintain the normal function of the inner ear and cardiac muscle.

2.1.3 X-linked SHL

Hearing loss conditions inherited with an X-linked pattern are rare. Only few syndromes with few patients were reported. Norrie disease and Mohr-Tranebjaerg syndrome are examples of X-Linked SHL.

Norrie disease is a rare X-linked recessive disorder characterized by progressive visual impairment. One-third of males with Norrie disease will develop progressive hearing loss and other phenotype-like intellectual disabilities. Mutation in *NDP* gene is the cause of 95% of the affected individuals. *NDP* is a gene that encodes Norrin protein which regulates vascularization of the retina [25].

Mohr-Tranebjaerg syndrome also called deafness dystonia optic atrophy syndrome is another X-linked recessive syndrome that is associated with early onset hearing loss, movement disability and visual impairment. Less than 70 cases of this syndrome were reported worldwide. *TIMM8A* is the causative gene for this syndrome which encodes the Translocase of Inner Mitochondrial Membrane 8 homolog A protein. This protein is important for the development of nervous system [26].

2.1.4 Mitochondrial-linked SHL

Maternally inherited diabetes and deafness (MIDD) is a mitochondrial disorder causing a syndromic form of diabetes accompanied by sensorineural hearing loss and some cases include renal problems, pigmentary retinopathy, ptosis, myopathy, cardiomyopathy and/or neuro-psychiatric symptoms (OMIM: 520000) [27, 28]. Mutations in MT-TL1, MT-TK or MT-TE mitochondrial genes coding for mtRNAs, which participate in the protein production in mitochondria and impair their functioning had been linked in MIDD [29].

2.2 Non-syndromic hearing loss

Hearing loss which is not associated with any other disease or symptoms is called non-syndromic hearing loss (NSHL). It accounts for more than 70% of hereditary hearing loss. According to the hereditary hearing loss homepage, there are more than 100 genes associated with NSHL and more than 6000 causative variants are identified so far which makes it extremely heterogeneous [30].

According to the mode of inheritance, NSHL can be classified as autosomal recessive (75–85%), autosomal dominant (20–25%) and X-linked or mitochondrial (1–2%). The loci responsible for NSHL are named DEN which stands for Deafness. Letter "A" is added, if the mode of inheritance is autosomal dominant (DFNA), "B" if the inheritance is recessive (DFNB) and "X" if the inheritance is X-linked (DFNX). The numbers indicate the chronological order of gene discovery.

2.2.1 Autosomal dominant NSHL genes (DFNA)

Autosomal dominant forms account for 20–25% of NSHL and are characterized by post-lingual progressive hearing loss [31]. More than 40 genes are associated with autosomal dominant NSHL. *DIAPH1* gene which is located in the DFNA1 locus is one of the first loci described for autosomal dominant NSHL. It encodes protein that is important for polymerization with actin which plays major role in cytoskeletal of hair cells in the inner ear. Mutations in *DIAPH1* are associated with early onset progressive hearing loss and some patients may have mild thrombocytopenia without bleeding tendencies [32].

WFS1 encodes for Wolframin protein which plays role in regulating cellular Ca_2^+ homeostasis and is involved in the process of sensory perception of sound. Mutations in *WFS1* are found to be associated with DFNA6, DFNA14 and DFNA38 in which they are characterized by hearing loss in low frequency [33, 34]. Some missense mutations in this gene are also associated with congenital profound hearing loss, progressive optic atrophy and diabetes. The above-mentioned phenotypes are a form of autosomal recessive hearing loss condition known as Wolfram syndrome [35].

The *TECTA* gene that encodes the tectorin-alpha protein forms the tectorial membrane in the cochlea and the otolithic membrane in the vestibular system. Mutations in *TECTA* are found in families with DFNA8/12 in which hearing loss could be pre- or post-lingual [36]. The severity of hearing loss varies depending on the domain where the mutation occurs. Some mutations in *TECTA* are also associated with DFNB21 hearing loss in which hearing loss is prelingual with severe to profound phenotype [37].

Deafness autosomal dominant 5 (*DFNA5*) gene that encodes for the Gasdermin-E protein is another gene associated with autosomal dominant non-syndromic hearing loss [38]. Gasdermin-E plays essential role in cellular response to DNA damage by regulating TP53.

Other genes associated with autosomal dominant hearing loss are listed in **Table 2**.

2.2.2 Autosomal recessive NSHL

Autosomal recessive hearing loss account for majority (75–85%) forms of non-syndromic hearing loss in which the hearing loss is prelingual and severe to profound. The most common gene causing autosomal recessive NSHL is *GJB2* accounts for 50% of the cases. The other 50% of the autosomal recessive NSHL resulted from mutations in 70 genes (**Table 2**).

Gene	Locus	OMIM entry	Inheritance
ACTG1	DFNA20/26	102560	AD
ADCY1	DFNB44	103072	AR
AIFM1	DFNX5	300169	XL
BDP1	DFNB49	607012	AR
BSND	DFNB73	606412	AR
CABP2	DFNB93	607314	AR
CCDC50	DFNA44	611051	AD
CD164	DFNA66	603356	AD
CDC14A	DFNB32/105	601728	AR
CDH23	DFNB12	605516	AR
CEACAM16	DFNA4B	614591	AD
CIB2	DFNB48	605564	AR
CLDN14	DFNB29	605608	AR
CLIC5	DFNB103	607293	AR
COCH	DFNA9	603196	AD
COL11A1	DFNA37	120280	AD
COL11A2	DFNB53, DFNA13	120290	AR, AD
COL4A6	DFNX6	303631	XL
CRYM	DFNA40	123740	AD
DCDC2	DFNB66	605755	AR
DIAPH1	DFNA1	602121	AD
DMXL2		612186	AD
ELMOD3	DFNB88	615427	AR
EPS8	DFNB102	600206	AR
EPS8L2	DFNB106	614988	AR
ESPN	DFNB36	606351	AR
ESRP1		609245	AR
ESRRB	DFNB35	602167	AR
EYA4	DFNA10	603550	AD
FAM65B	DFNB104	611410	AR
GIPC3	DFNB15/72/95	608792	AR
GJB2	DFNB1A, DFNA3A	121011	AR, AD
GJB3	DFNA2B	603324	AD
GJB6	DFNB1B, DFNA3B	604418	AR, AD
GPSM2	DFNB82	609245	AR
GRHL2	DFNA28	608576	AD
GRXCR1	DFNB25	613283	AR
GRXCR2	DFNB101	615762	AR
GSDME/DFNA5	DFNA5	608798	AD
HGF	DFNB39	142409	AR
HOMER2	DFNA68	604799	AD
IFNLR1	DFNA2C	607404	AD
ILDR1	DFNB42	609739	AR

Gene	Locus	OMIM entry	Inheritance
KARS	DFNB89	601421	AR
KCNQ4	DFNA2A	603537	AD
KITLG	DFNA69	184745	AD
LHFPL5	DFNB66/67	609427	AR
LMX1A	DFNA7	600298	AD
LOXHD1	DFNB77	613072	AR
LRTOMT/COMT2	DFNB63	612414	AR
MARVELD2	DFNB49	610572	AR
MCM2	DFNA70	116945	AD
MET	DFNB97	164860	AR
MIRN96	DFNA50	611606	AD
MPZL2		604873	AR
MSRB3	DFNB74	613719	AR
MTRNR1		561000	MIT
MTTS1		590080	MIT
MYH14	DFNA4A	608568	AD
MYH9	DFNA17	160775	AD
MYO15A	DFNB3	602666	AR
MYO3A	DFNB30	606808	AR, AD
MYO6	DFNB37, DFNA22	600970	AR, AD
MYO7A	DFNB2, DFNA11	276903	AR, AD
NARS2	DFNB94	612803	AR
NLRP3	DFNA34	606416	AD
OSBPL2	DFNA67	606731	AD
OTOA	DFNB22	607038	AR
OTOF	DFNB9	603681	AR
OTOG	DFNB18B	604487	AR
OTOGL	DFNB84	614925	AR
P2RX2	DFNA41	600844	AD
PCDH15	DFNB23	605514	AR
PDE1C		602987	AD
PDZD7	DFNB57	612971	AR
PJVK	DFNB59	610219	AR
PNPT1	DFNB70	610316	AR
POU3F4	DFNX2	300039	XL
POU4F3	DFNA15	602460	AD
PPIP5K2	DFNB100	611648	AR
PRPS1	DFNX1	311850	XL
PTPRQ	DFNB84, DFNA73	603317	AR, AD
RDX	DFNB24	179410	AR
REST	DFNA27	600571	AD
ROR1	DFNB108	612959	AR
S1PR2	DFNB68	609427	AR
SERPINB6	DFNB91	173321	AR

Gene	Locus	OMIM entry	Inheritance
SIX1	DFNA23	601205	AD
SLC17A8	DFNA25	607557	AD
SLC22A4	DFNB60	604943	AR
SLC26A4	DFNB4	605646	AR
SLC26A5	DFNB61	604943	AR
SMAC/DIABLO	DFNA64	605219	AD
SMPX	DFNX4	300226	XL
STRC	DFNB16	606440	AR
SYNE4	DFNB76	615535	AR
TBC1D24	DFNB86, DFNA65	613577	AR, AD
TECTA	DFNB21, DFNA8/12	602574	AR, AD
TJP2	DFNA51	607709	AD
TMC1	DFNB7/11, DFNA36	606706	AR, AD
TMEM132E	DFNB99	616178	AR
TMIE	DFNB6	607237	AR
TMPRSS3	DFNB8/10	605511	AR
TNC	DFNA56	187380	AD
TPRN	DFNB79	613354	AR
TRIOBP	DFNB28	609761	AR
TSPEAR	DFNB98	612920	AR
Unknown	DFNY1	400043	YL
USH1C	DFNB18	605242	AR
WBP2		606962	AR
WFS1	DFNA6/14/38	606201	AD
WHRN	DFNB31	607928	AR

Table 2.
List of genes associated with autosomal dominant (AD), autosomal recessive (AR), X-linked (XL) and mitochondrial (MIT) non-syndromic hearing loss (NSHL) [12].

GJB2 gene is one of the gap junction proteins that are expressed in the inner ear, which encodes connexin 26. This protein allows the exchange of potassium ions between the cells in the inner ear. More than 100 mutations identified in *GJB2* were found to cause DFNB1 and DFNA3 [39].

Other gene related to *GJB2* is *GJB6* that encodes for connexin 30 protein. Studies show that both genes can be inherited together and 8% of patients with *GJB2* mutation also carry mutation in *GJB6* [40].

OTOF gene encodes otoferlin protein that is responsible for the neural transmission at the synaptic cleft of the inner hair cell. Mutations in this gene cause prelingual, profound autosomal recessive hearing loss (DFNB9) and will result in damage of the neural receptors of the inner ear that will result on interruption of the nerve pathways to the brain [41].

Conventional and unconventional myosins are group of genes that are functioning as actin-binding proteins. Conventional myosins regulate contractility of actin filaments, while unconventional myosins are essential for vesicle trafficking and endocytosis [42]. Mutations in some unconventional myosins are associated with NSHL. *MYO6* is an example of unconventional myosins that is expressed in the inner hair cell of the cochlea. Mutation in *MYO6* causes DFNB37, a form of non-syndromic deafness characterized by prelingual severe to profound hearing loss [43]. Other genes are listed in **Table 2**.

2.2.3 X-linked NSHL

This form of hearing loss is very rare and only few genes are associated with non-syndromic hearing loss (**Table 2**). This form of hearing loss is characterized by progressive, conductive and sensorineural hearing loss. Mutations in *POU3F4* gene which cause DFNX2, account for 50% of the cases [44]. *POU3F4* gene encode for POU domain class 3 transcription factor 4 protein, which regulates the proliferation of neural cells in middle and inner ear early during development. Because this form of hearing loss is X-linked, the severity of hearing loss differs from male to female. In males, hearing loss is prelingual and range from severe to profound while in females hearing loss is post-lingual and less severe.

2.2.4 Mitochondrial-linked NSHL

Despite the crucial role of mitochondria producing the energy for the cell, there are mtDNA mutations which lead to non-syndromic hearing impairment. The carriers exhibited sensorineural hearing loss with variable severity and onset [45]. These mutations have been reported in the mitochondrial genes encoding for 12S rRNA and tRNA genes [46, 47].

2.3 Age-related hearing loss

The auditory system exhibits senescent changes with the past time which could trigger to acquire sensorineural hearing loss. The most of acquired-hearing loss are characterized by a bilateral inner ear degeneration determined by genetic factors superimposed with environmental stress [48], excluding injuries and severe infections. Noise, drugs, aging and/or other systemic conditions (i.e., diabetes or hypertension [49, 50]) are numerous variables that can contribute to the final outcome of the disease [51, 52]. It is habitual among the causes of life related hearing loss that the severity progress beginning as mild loss and worsening over time.

The noise-induced hearing loss (NIHL) is one of the most common work-related diseases caused by the extreme exposure to noise. Recurrent exposure to noise causes physical damage to hair cells in the cochlea. Moreover, genetic predisposition and systemic conditions also contribute to the prevalence and severity of the phenotype making it difficult to distinguish the cause [53]. In the same line, there is a correlation between hazardous daily noise exposure and the prevalence of hearing loss among youth population [54, 55].

Ototoxic agents like certain drugs or heavy metals could contribute to the development of hearing impairment. Drugs such as cisplatin and aminoglycoside trigger hair cells apoptosis by enhancing the production of oxygen reactivity spices and has up to 50% reported incidence of irreversible hearing loss [56, 57].

The age-related hearing loss (ARHL) or presbycusis is caused by progressive atrophy of the inner ear during aging [58, 59]. The onset and prevalence of the disease vary widely as is multifactorial and many components (genetic and environmental) could play a role. Moreover, the heritability of AHRL had been stablished around 50% [60–64] and through genome-wide association studies and animal models, several age-related hearing loss genes had been identified [65–67]. The estimated prevalence of ARHL is one-third of adults above 65 years old and it doubles by each decade of life span [68, 69].

ARHL had been well-documented during the years because of its high prevalence in the population. Characterized cochlea manly by atrophy in the basal turns of the cochlea and is manifested by abrupt high-tone hearing loss [70, 71]. ARHL is commonly classified as sensory, neural and metabolic. Sensory ARHL stems from the progressive degeneration of organ of Corti [72], neural ARHL is considered when there is 50% or more of cochlear neurons loss [73] and metabolic ARHL is

Gene	Gene name	Phenotype	Study	Ref.
APOE	Apolipoprotein E	undefined	GWAS	[79]
ARHI	Age-related Hearing Loss	SN, M	GWAS	[80–82]
CDH23	Cadherin-related 23	SN, M	Model, GWAS	[83–86]
COX 3	cytochrome c oxidase subunit 3	M	Model	[87, 88]
EDN1	Endothelin-1	M	Model, GWAS	[89, 90]
GRHL2	Grainyhead-like 2	SN	GWAS	[91]
GRM7	Metabotropic glutamate receptor type 7	SN	GWAS	[92]
GST	Glutathione S-transferase	M	Model, GWAS	[93–95]
IQGAP2	IQ motif containing GTPase activating protein 2	undefined	GWAS	[96, 97]
ITGA8	Integrin, alpha 8	SN	Model	[98, 99]
KCNMA1	Potassium large conductance calcium-activated channel, subfamily M, alpha member 1	SN	Model	[100]
KCNQ1	Potassium voltage-gated channel, KQT-like subfamily, member 1	SN	GWAS	[101, 102]
KCNQ4	Potassium voltage-gated channel, KQT-like subfamily, member 4	SN, M	Model, GWAS	[103, 104]
NAT2	N-acetyltransferase 2	M	GWAS	[105–107]
P2X	Ligand-gated ion channel purinergic receptor 2	undefined	GWAS	[108]
PCDH15	Protocadherin-related 15	SN	Model, GWAS	[109, 110]
PTPRD	tyrosine phosphatase, receptor type D	undefined	GWAS	[111]
SLC26A4	Solute carrier family 26 member 4	SN	Model	[112]
SLC7A8	Solute carrier family 7 member 8	SN, M	Model, GWAS	[67]
SLC9A3R1	Regulator 1 of SLC9 transporter	SN	Model, GWAS	[113]
SPATC1L	Spermatogenesis and centriole associated 1	undefined	GWAS	[114]
SPNS2	Spinster homolog 2	M	Model	[115, 116]
TBL1Y	Transducin beta-like 1 Y-linked	SN	Model, GWAS	[117]
THRB	Thyroid hormone receptor 1	SN, M	Model, GWAS	[118]
TNF	Tumor necrosis factor	M	GWAS	[119]
UCP2	Uncoupling protein 2	SN	GWAS	[120, 121]

Inner ear phenotype classification: sensorineural (SN), metabolic (M) and both of them (SN and M). Study type: genome-wide association study and study-case (GWAS) and in vitro or in vivo model (Model).

Table 3.
ARHL-related genes.

caused by the atrophy of the stria vascularis resulting in a decrease in endolymphatic potential [74]. Also, there is a mixed type where the progressive degeneration of sensory cells is observed along loss of cochlear neurons [75–77]. Moreover, still controversial if the loss of neurons is a secondary consequence or a primary cause.

The task to distinct between genetic and environmental factors in acquired hearing loss is very challenging. In this regard, to progress the understanding of the mechanisms that lead to the damage, physiopathology of age-related hearing loss had been assessed by *in vitro* (cell lines) and *in vivo* (rodents and zebrafish) models [70]. The studies provided evidences of specific inner damage such as inflammation, oxidative stress, reduced cochlear blood flow, disrupted ion hemostasis and death of sensory and neuronal cells [78]. **Table 3** summarizes all current knowledge on ARHL-related genetic factors.

2.3.1 Consequences of suffering ARHL

Age-related hearing loss affects communication and information reception reducing the quality of live and psychosocial well-being (e.g., anxiety or depression) of elder population. Limitation in communication has an impact on social and personal relationships triggering to loss of autonomy and dependency [122, 123]. Even though the World Health Organization estimates that by 2025 approximately 500 million will suffer from age-related hearing loss; there is a lack of awareness by health care professionals as well as no educational programs on how patients could overcome obstacles caused by hearing loss.

Few studies have investigated the psychological factor and how individuals develop their lives in the presence of hearing loss. The studies reveal that maladaptive behavior (e.g., escape, avoiding social interaction and/or pretending to understand) has a negative effect on well-being of elder patients comparing to adaptive strategies (e.g., training verbal skills or self-awareness) [124, 125]. Additionally, there is a significant increase of hearing aids use by cases who attend audiology clinic with a relative than others attending alone [126]. Therefore, elder population with acquired hearing loss requires social support from family and health care professionals. Educational programs on how to use hearing aids and communication strategies as well as counseling for follow-up and feedback are needed in order to increase adherence to treatment and improve life quality [127].

3. Hearing loss treatments

Hearing loss is not a curable disease however science made some considerable progress. Current therapies based on cochlear implants (a device that provides direct electrical stimulation to the auditory nerve in the inner ear) and hearing aids (are non-surgically placed in the ear canal) which help patients to recover partly hearing.

Hearing aids could be a stigma in the society as are negatively perceived as well as expensive making that only one out of five people who could benefit from a hearing aid actually wears it (WHO, [128]). Therefore, the major barriers to improve hearing in elder population include perception that hearing loss is a normal part of aging or is not amenable to treatment.

Based on the animal research studies, several clinical trials are working to investigate the effects of a variety of drugs to prevent hearing loss including antioxidants, ROS scavengers, alpha lipoic acid, N-acetylcysteine or anti-inflammatory agents [129–134].

New generation treatments based on microRNA, short interfering RNA as well as tissue regeneration using stem cells are promising tools [135, 136]. Due to the in-depth study of stem cell and its therapeutic potential, stem cell technology opened new approaches for hair cell and auditory nerve regeneration [137, 138]. By using two strategies of endogenous stem cell activation and exogenous stem cell transplantation, exciting results on restoring hearing function are showed. Even though the use of stem cells to repair cochlear injury is relatively new, they appear to be a very promising possibility for the treatment of hearing loss induced by noise, aging or ototoxic drugs. These three causes comprise a major part of the burden of hearing loss, so if this approach were successful could have a large public health effect of hearing impairment. Further research should be supported to solve the problems which limit stem cells application in humans.

4. Conclusion

Of the senses that humans use to interact with their environment, hearing is considered as one of the dominant after vision. The loss of hearing can occur through genetic mutations, through environmental factors or through a combination of both. ARHL is an increasingly important public health problem which reduces life's quality, isolation, dependence and frustration. Besides basic research and more effective therapies for the optimal treatment, management of the condition is still a pending task. Social support by the family and health care professionals is critical to the life quality of the older adults with hearing loss. The quality of care and well-being could be improved by active education and counseling to provide appropriate support to facilitate everyday communication.

Acknowledgements

Meritxell Espino-Guarch received funding from Qatar Foundation Grant ID: JSREP07-03-3-006.

Conflict of interest

There is no conflict of interest.

Author details

Moza Al-Kowari* and Meritxell Espino-Guarch
Translational Medicine, Sidra Medicine Hospital, Doha, Qatar

*Address all correspondence to: malkowari@sidra.org

References

[1] Duthey B. Hearing Loss. WHO; 2018. Available from: https://www.who.int/news-room/fact-sheets/detail/deafness-and-hearing-loss

[2] Sanchez-Calderon H, Rodriguez-de la Rosa L, Milo M, Pichel JG, Holley M, Varela-Nieto I. RNA microarray analysis in prenatal mouse cochlea reveals novel IGF-I target genes: Implication of MEF2 and FOXM1 transcription factors. PLoS One. 2010;**5**(1):e8699

[3] Zahnert T. The differential diagnosis of hearing loss. Deutsches Ärzteblatt International. 2011;**108**(25):433-443. quiz 44

[4] Wilson WR, Byl FM, Laird N. The efficacy of steroids in the treatment of idiopathic sudden hearing loss. A double-blind clinical study. Archives of Otolaryngology. 1980;**106**(12):772-776

[5] Lee JH, Lee MY, Lim Y, Knowles J, Kim HW. Auditory disorders and future therapies with delivery systems. Journal of Tissue Engineering. 2018;**9**:2041731418808455

[6] Angeli S, Lin X, Liu XZ. Genetics of hearing and deafness. Anatomical Record (Hoboken). 2012;**295**(11):1812-1829

[7] Cruickshanks KJ, Nondahl DM, Tweed TS, Wiley TL, Klein BE, Klein R, et al. Education, occupation, noise exposure history and the 10-yr cumulative incidence of hearing impairment in older adults. Hearing Research. 2010;**264**(1-2):3-9

[8] Christensen K, Frederiksen H, Hoffman HJ. Genetic and environmental influences on self-reported reduced hearing in the old and oldest old. Journal of the American Geriatrics Society. 2001;**49**(11):1512-1517

[9] Smith RJ, Bale JF, White KR. Sensorineural hearing loss in children. Lancet. 2005;**365**(9462):879-890

[10] Bork JM, Peters LM, Riazuddin S, Bernstein SL, Ahmed ZM, Ness SL, et al. Usher syndrome 1D and nonsyndromic autosomal recessive deafness DFNB12 are caused by allelic mutations of the novel cadherin-like gene CDH23. American Journal of Human Genetics. 2001;**68**(1):26-37

[11] Waardenburg PJ. A new syndrome combining developmental anomalies of the eyelids, eyebrows and nose root with pigmentary defects of the iris and head hair and with congenital deafness. American Journal of Human Genetics. 1951;**3**(3):195-253

[12] Hereditary Hearing Loss Homepage. 2018. Available from: https://hereditaryhearingloss.org/

[13] Smith RJH. Branchiootorenal spectrum disorder. In: Adam MP, Ardinger HH, Pagon RA, Wallace SE, LJH B, Stephens K, et al., editors. GeneReviews((R)). Seattle (WA): University of Washington, Seattle University of Washington, Seattle; 1993. GeneReviews is a registered trademark of the University of Washington, Seattle. All rights reserved.

[14] Martin DM. Epigenetic developmental disorders: CHARGE syndrome, a case study. Current Genetic Medicine Reports. 2015;**3**(1):1-7

[15] Vernon M. Usher's syndrome—Deafness and progressive blindness. Clinical cases, prevention, theory and literature survey. Journal of Chronic Diseases. 1969;**22**(3):133-151

[16] Furth ED, Carvalho M, Vianna B. Familial goiter due to an organification defect in euthyroid siblings. Journal of Clinical

Endocrinology and Metabolism. 1967;**27**(8):1137-1140

[17] Reardon W, Trembath RC. Pendred syndrome. Journal of Medical Genetics. 1996;**33**(12):1037-1040

[18] Pourová R, Janousek P, Jurovcík M, Dvoráková M, Malíková M, Rasková D, et al. Spectrum and frequency of SLC26A4 mutations among Czech patients with early hearing loss with and without enlarged vestibular aqueduct (EVA). Annals of Human Genetics. 2010;**74**(4):299-307

[19] Yang T, Vidarsson H, Rodrigo-Blomqvist S, Rosengren SS, Enerback S, Smith RJ. Transcriptional control of SLC26A4 is involved in Pendred syndrome and nonsyndromic enlargement of vestibular aqueduct (DFNB4). American Journal of Human Genetics. 2007;**80**(6):1055-1063

[20] Yang T, Gurrola JG, Wu H, Chiu SM, Wangemann P, Snyder PM, et al. Mutations of KCNJ10 together with mutations of SLC26A4 cause digenic nonsyndromic hearing loss associated with enlarged vestibular aqueduct syndrome. American Journal of Human Genetics. 2009;**84**(5):651-657

[21] Jervell A, Lange-Nielsen F. Congenital deaf mutism, functional heart disease with prolongation of the Q-T interval and sudden death. American Heart Journal. 1957;**54**(1):59-68

[22] Koffler T, Ushakov K, Avraham KB. Genetics of hearing loss: Syndromic. Otolaryngologic Clinics of North America. 2015;**48**(6):1041-1061

[23] Neyroud N, Tesson F, Denjoy I, Leibovici M, Donger C, Barhanin J, et al. A novel mutation in the potassium channel gene KVLQT1 causes the Jervell and Lange-Nielsen cardioauditory syndrome. Nature Genetics. 1997;**15**(2):186-189

[24] Schulze-Bahr E, Wang Q, Wedekind H, Haverkamp W, Chen Q, Sun Y, et al. KCNE1 mutations cause jervell and Lange-Nielsen syndrome. Nature Genetics. 1997;**17**(3):267-268

[25] Berger W, van de Pol D, Warburg M, Gal A, Bleeker-Wagemakers L, de Silva H, et al. Mutations in the candidate gene for Norrie disease. Human Molecular Genetics. 1992;**1**(7):461-465

[26] Roesch K, Hynds PJ, Varga R, Tranebjaerg L, Koehler CM. The calcium-binding aspartate/glutamate carriers, citrin and aralar1, are new substrates for the DDP1/TIMM8a-TIMM13 complex. Human Molecular Genetics. 2004;**13**(18):2101-2111

[27] Li HZ, Li RY, Li M. A review of maternally inherited diabetes and deafness. Frontiers in Bioscience (Landmark Edition). 2014;**19**:777-782

[28] Naing A, Kenchaiah M, Krishnan B, Mir F, Charnley A, Egan C, et al. Maternally inherited diabetes and deafness (MIDD): Diagnosis and management. Journal of Diabetes and Its Complications. 2014;**28**(4):542-546

[29] Tabebi M, Charfi N, Kallabi F, Alila-Fersi O, Ben Mahmoud A, Tlili A, et al. Whole mitochondrial genome screening of a family with maternally inherited diabetes and deafness (MIDD) associated with retinopathy: A putative haplotype associated to MIDD and a novel MT-CO2 m.8241T>G mutation. Journal of Diabetes and its Complications. 2017;**31**(1):253-259

[30] Sloan-Heggen CM, Smith RJ. Navigating genetic diagnostics in patients with hearing loss. Current Opinion in Pediatrics. 2016;**28**(6):705-712

[31] Taylor KR, Deluca AP, Shearer AE, Hildebrand MS, Black-Ziegelbein EA, Anand VN, et al. AudioGene: Predicting hearing loss genotypes from phenotypes

to guide genetic screening. Human Mutation. 2013;**34**(4):539-545

[32] Neuhaus C, Lang-Roth R, Zimmermann U, Heller R, Eisenberger T, Weikert M, et al. Extension of the clinical and molecular phenotype of DIAPH1-associated autosomal dominant hearing loss (DFNA1). Clinical Genetics. 2017;**91**(6):892-901

[33] Bespalova IN, Van Camp G, Bom SJ, Brown DJ, Cryns K, DeWan AT, et al. Mutations in the Wolfram syndrome 1 gene (WFS1) are a common cause of low frequency sensorineural hearing loss. Human Molecular Genetics. 2001;**10**(22):2501-2508

[34] Young TL, Ives E, Lynch E, Person R, Snook S, MacLaren L, et al. Non-syndromic progressive hearing loss DFNA38 is caused by heterozygous missense mutation in the Wolfram syndrome gene WFS1. Human Molecular Genetics. 2001;**10**(22):2509-2514

[35] Cryns K, Sivakumaran TA, Van den Ouweland JM, Pennings RJ, Cremers CW, Flothmann K, et al. Mutational spectrum of the WFS1 gene in Wolfram syndrome, nonsyndromic hearing impairment, diabetes mellitus, and psychiatric disease. Human Mutation. 2003;**22**(4):275-287

[36] Verhoeven K, Van Laer L, Kirschhofer K, Legan PK, Hughes DC, Schatteman I, et al. Mutations in the human alpha-tectorin gene cause autosomal dominant non-syndromic hearing impairment. Nature Genetics. 1998;**19**(1):60-62

[37] Mustapha M, Weil D, Chardenoux S, Elias S, El-Zir E, Beckmann JS, et al. An alpha-tectorin gene defect causes a newly identified autosomal recessive form of sensorineural pre-lingual non-syndromic deafness, DFNB21. Human Molecular Genetics. 1999;**8**(3):409-412

[38] Van Laer L, Huizing EH, Verstreken M, van Zuijlen D, Wauters JG, Bossuyt PJ, et al. Nonsyndromic hearing impairment is associated with a mutation in DFNA5. Nature Genetics. 1998;**20**(2):194-197

[39] Kelsell DP, Dunlop J, Stevens HP, Lench NJ, Liang JN, Parry G, et al. Connexin 26 mutations in hereditary non-syndromic sensorineural deafness. Nature. 1997;**387**(6628):80-83

[40] Venkatesh MD, Moorchung N, Puri B. Genetics of non syndromic hearing loss. Medical Journal Armed Forces India. 2015;**71**(4):363-368

[41] Yasunaga S, Grati M, Cohen-Salmon M, El-Amraoui A, Mustapha M, Salem N, et al. A mutation in OTOF, encoding otoferlin, a FER-1-like protein, causes DFNB9, a nonsyndromic form of deafness. Nature Genetics. 1999;**21**(4):363-369

[42] Duman D, Tekin M. Autosomal recessive nonsyndromic deafness genes: A review. Frontiers in Bioscience (Landmark Edition). 2012;**17**:2213-2236

[43] Ahmed ZM, Morell RJ, Riazuddin S, Gropman A, Shaukat S, Ahmad MM, et al. Mutations of MYO6 are associated with recessive deafness, DFNB37. American Journal of Human Genetics. 2003;**72**(5):1315-1322

[44] de Kok YJ, van der Maarel SM, Bitner-Glindzicz M, Huber I, Monaco AP, Malcolm S, et al. Association between X-linked mixed deafness and mutations in the POU domain gene POU3F4. Science. 1995;**267**(5198):685-688

[45] Van Camp G, Smith RJ. Maternally inherited hearing impairment. Clinical Genetics. 2000;**57**(6):409-414

[46] Moassass F, Al-Halabi B, Nweder MS, Al-Achkar W. Investigation of the mtDNA mutations in Syrian families

with non-syndromic sensorineural hearing loss. International Journal of Pediatric Otorhinolaryngology. 2018;**113**:110-114

[47] Chen X, Nie Z, Wang F, Wang J, Liu XW, Zheng J, et al. Late onset nonsyndromic hearing loss in a Dongxiang Chinese family is associated with the 593T>C variant in the mitochondrial tRNA. Mitochondrion. 2017;**35**:111-118

[48] Howarth A, Shone GR. Ageing and the auditory system. Postgraduate Medical Journal. 2006;**82**(965):166-171

[49] Cruickshanks KJ, Dhar S, Dinces E, Fifer RC, Gonzalez F, Heiss G, et al. Hearing impairment prevalence and associated risk factors in the hispanic community health study/study of Latinos. JAMA Otolaryngology. Head and Neck Surgery. 2015;**141**(7):641-648

[50] Cruickshanks KJ, Nondahl DM, Dalton DS, Fischer ME, Klein BE, Klein R, et al. Smoking, central adiposity, and poor glycemic control increase risk of hearing impairment. Journal of the American Geriatrics Society. 2015;**63**(5):918-924

[51] Bovo R, Ciorba A, Martini A. Environmental and genetic factors in age-related hearing impairment. Aging Clinical and Experimental Research. 2011;**23**(1):3-10

[52] Momi SK, Wolber LE, Fabiane SM, MacGregor AJ, Williams FM. Genetic and environmental factors in age-related hearing impairment. Twin Research and Human Genetics. 2015;**18**(4):383-392

[53] Attias J, Horovitz G, El-Hatib N, Nageris B. Detection and clinical diagnosis of noise-induced hearing loss by otoacoustic emissions. Noise and Health. 2001;**3**(12):19-31

[54] Shargorodsky J, Curhan SG, Curhan GC, Eavey R. Change in prevalence of hearing loss in US adolescents. Journal of the American Medical Association. 2010;**304**(7):772-778

[55] Henderson E, Testa MA, Hartnick C. Prevalence of noise-induced hearing-threshold shifts and hearing loss among US youths. Pediatrics. 2011;**127**(1):e39-e46

[56] Callejo A, Sedó-Cabezón L, Juan ID, Llorens J. Cisplatin-induced ototoxicity: Effects, mechanisms and protection strategies. Toxics. 2015;**3**(3):268-293

[57] Jiang M, Karasawa T, Steyger PS. Aminoglycoside-induced cochleotoxicity: A review. Frontiers in Cellular Neuroscience. 2017;**11**:308

[58] McGill TJ, Schuknecht HF. Human cochlear changes in noise induced hearing loss. The Laryngoscope. 1976;**86**(9):1293-1302

[59] Liu XZ, Yan D. Ageing and hearing loss. Journal of Pathology. 2007;**211**(2):188-197

[60] Wingfield A, Panizzon M, Grant MD, Toomey R, Kremen WS, Franz CE, et al. A twin-study of genetic contributions to hearing acuity in late middle age. The Journals of Gerontology. Series A, Biological Sciences and Medical Sciences. 2007;**62**(11):1294-1299

[61] Cruickshanks KJ, Klein R, Klein BE, Nondahl DM. Sunlight and the 5-year incidence of early age-related maculopathy: The beaver dam eye study. Archives of Ophthalmology. 2001;**119**(2):246-250

[62] Gates GA, Couropmitree NN, Myers RH. Genetic associations in age-related hearing thresholds. Archives of Otolaryngology—Head and Neck Surgery. 1999;**125**(6):654-659

[63] Karlsson KK, Harris JR, Svartengren M. Description and

primary results from an audiometric study of male twins. Ear and Hearing. 1997;**18**(2):114-120

[64] Cruickshanks KJ, Wiley TL, Tweed TS, Klein BE, Klein R, Mares-Perlman JA, et al. Prevalence of hearing loss in older adults in beaver dam, Wisconsin. The epidemiology of hearing loss study. American Journal of Epidemiology. 1998;**148**(9):879-886

[65] Payton PDaA. Genetics of age-related hearing loss. Genetics of Deafness. 2016;**20**:84-96

[66] Van Eyken E, Van Camp G, Van Laer L. The complexity of age-related hearing impairment: Contributing environmental and genetic factors. Audiology and Neuro-Otology. 2007;**12**(6):345-358

[67] Espino Guarch M, Font-Llitjós M, Murillo-Cuesta S, Errasti-Murugarren E, Celaya AM, Girotto G, et al. Mutations in L-type amino acid transporter-2 support. eLife. 2018;**7**

[68] Lin FR. Hearing loss and cognition among older adults in the United States. The Journals of Gerontology. Series A, Biological Sciences and Medical Sciences. 2011;**66**(10):1131-1136

[69] Lin FR, Thorpe R, Gordon-Salant S, Ferrucci L. Hearing loss prevalence and risk factors among older adults in the United States. The Journals of Gerontology. Series A, Biological Sciences and Medical Sciences. 2011;**66**(5):582-590

[70] Fetoni AR, Picciotti PM, Paludetti G, Troiani D. Pathogenesis of presbycusis in animal models: A review. Experimental Gerontology. 2011;**46**(6):413-425

[71] Lee KY. Pathophysiology of age-related hearing loss (peripheral and central). Korean Journal of Audiology. 2013;**17**(2):45-49

[72] Schuknecht HF, Gacek MR. Cochlear pathology in presbycusis. The Annals of Otology, Rhinology, and Laryngology. 1993;**102**(1 Pt 2):1-16

[73] Makary CA, Shin J, Kujawa SG, Liberman MC, Merchant SN. Age-related primary cochlear neuronal degeneration in human temporal bones. Journal of the Association for Research in Otolaryngology. 2011;**12**(6):711-717

[74] Pauler M, Schuknecht HF, White JA. Atrophy of the stria vascularis as a cause of sensorineural hearing loss. The Laryngoscope. 1988;**98**(7):754-759

[75] Stankovic K, Rio C, Xia A, Sugawara M, Adams JC, Liberman MC, et al. Survival of adult spiral ganglion neurons requires erbB receptor signaling in the inner ear. Journal of Neuroscience. 2004;**24**(40):8651-8661

[76] Sugawara M, Murtie JC, Stankovic KM, Liberman MC, Corfas G. Dynamic patterns of neurotrophin 3 expression in the postnatal mouse inner ear. Journal of Comparative Neurology. 2007;**501**(1):30-37

[77] Zilberstein Y, Liberman MC, Corfas G. Inner hair cells are not required for survival of spiral ganglion neurons in the adult cochlea. Journal of Neuroscience. 2012;**32**(2):405-410

[78] Castañeda R, Natarajan S, Jeong SY, Hong BN, Kang TH. Traditional oriental medicine for sensorineural hearing loss: Can ethnopharmacology contribute to potential drug discovery? Journal of Ethnopharmacology. 2018;**231**:409-428

[79] O'Grady G, Boyles AL, Speer M, DeRuyter F, Strittmatter W, Worley G. Apolipoprotein E alleles and sensorineural hearing loss. International Journal of Audiology. 2007;**46**(4):183-186

[80] Johnson KR, Erway LC, Cook SA, Willott JF, Zheng QY. A major gene

affecting age-related hearing loss in C57BL/6J mice. Hearing Research. 1997;**114**(1-2):83-92

[81] DeStefano AL, Gates GA, Heard-Costa N, Myers RH, Baldwin CT. Genomewide linkage analysis to presbycusis in the Framingham Heart Study. Archives of Otolaryngology—Head and Neck Surgery. 2003;**129**(3):285-289

[82] Garringer HJ, Pankratz ND, Nichols WC, Reed T. Hearing impairment susceptibility in elderly men and the DFNA18 locus. Archives of Otolaryngology—Head and Neck Surgery. 2006;**132**(5):506-510

[83] Di Palma F, Pellegrino R, Noben-Trauth K. Genomic structure, alternative splice forms and normal and mutant alleles of cadherin 23 (Cdh23). Gene. 2001;**281**(1-2):31-41

[84] Noben-Trauth K, Zheng QY, Johnson KR. Association of cadherin 23 with polygenic inheritance and genetic modification of sensorineural hearing loss. Nature Genetics. 2003;**35**(1):21-23

[85] Davis RR, Kozel P, Erway LC. Genetic influences in individual susceptibility to noise: A review. Noise and Health. 2003;**5**(20):19-28

[86] Liu S, Li S, Zhu H, Cheng S, Zheng QY. A mutation in the cdh23 gene causes age-related hearing loss in Cdh23(nmf308/nmf308) mice. Gene. 2012;**499**(2):309-317

[87] Markaryan A, Nelson EG, Hinojosa R. Quantification of the mitochondrial DNA common deletion in presbycusis. The Laryngoscope. 2009;**119**(6):1184-1189

[88] Markaryan A, Nelson EG, Hinojosa R. Major arc mitochondrial DNA deletions in cytochrome c oxidase-deficient human cochlear spiral ganglion cells. Acta Oto-Laryngologica. 2010;**130**(7):780-787

[89] Uchida Y, Sugiura S, Nakashima T, Ando F, Shimokata H. Endothelin-1 gene polymorphism and hearing impairment in elderly Japanese. The Laryngoscope. 2009;**119**(5):938-943

[90] Xu D, Tang Y, Liu S, Liu J. Expression and significance of endothelin 1 in spiral ganglion cells of guinea pig. International Journal of Pediatric Otorhinolaryngology. 2008;**72**(2):189-192

[91] Van Laer L, Van Eyken E, Fransen E, Huyghe JR, Topsakal V, Hendrickx JJ, et al. The grainyhead like 2 gene (GRHL2), alias TFCP2L3, is associated with age-related hearing impairment. Human Molecular Genetics. 2008;**17**(2):159-169

[92] Friedman RA, Van Laer L, Huentelman MJ, Sheth SS, Van Eyken E, Corneveaux JJ, et al. GRM7 variants confer susceptibility to age-related hearing impairment. Human Molecular Genetics. 2009;**18**(4):785-796

[93] Bared A, Ouyang X, Angeli S, Du LL, Hoang K, Yan D, et al. Antioxidant enzymes, presbycusis, and ethnic variability. Otolaryngology and Head and Neck Surgery. 2010;**143**(2):263-268

[94] Takumi Y, Matsubara A, Tsuchida S, Ottersen OP, Shinkawa H, Usami S. Various glutathione S-transferase isoforms in the rat cochlea. Neuroreport. 2001;**12**(7):1513-1516

[95] Ateş NA, Unal M, Tamer L, Derici E, Karakaş S, Ercan B, et al. Glutathione S-transferase gene polymorphisms in presbycusis. Otology and Neurotology. 2005;**26**(3):392-397

[96] Luo H, Wu H, Shen H, Chen H, Yang T, Huang Z, et al. The European GWAS-identified risk SNP rs457717 within IQGAP2 is not associated with age-related hearing impairment in Han male Chinese population. European Archives of Oto-Rhino-Laryngology. 2016;**273**(7):1677-1687

[97] Van Laer L, Huyghe JR, Hannula S, Van Eyken E, Stephan DA, Mäki-Torkko E, et al. A genome-wide association study for age-related hearing impairment in the Saami. European Journal of Human Genetics. 2010;**18**(6):685-693

[98] Goodman L, Zallocchi M. Integrin α8 and Pcdh15 act as a complex to regulate cilia biogenesis in sensory cells. Journal of Cell Science. 2017;**130**(21):3698-3712

[99] Li F, Zhuang J, Chen Y, Gao B, Gu H, Zhou X. Difference of cervical vestibular evoked myogenic potentials in different audition stage of Ménière disease. Lin Chuang Er Bi Yan Hou Tou Jing Wai Ke Za Zhi. 2016;**30**(1):9-12

[100] Rüttiger L, Sausbier M, Zimmermann U, Winter H, Braig C, Engel J, et al. Deletion of the Ca^{2+}-activated potassium (BK) alpha-subunit but not the BKbeta1-subunit leads to progressive hearing loss. Proceedings of the National Academy of Sciences of the United States of America. 2004;**101**(35):12922-12927

[101] Wasano K, Mutai H, Obuchi C, Masuda S, Matsunaga T. A novel frameshift mutation in KCNQ4 in a family with autosomal recessive non-syndromic hearing loss. Biochemical and Biophysical Research Communications. 2015;**463**(4):582-586

[102] Xiong H, Chu H, Zhou X, Huang X, Cui Y, Zhou L, et al. Simultaneously reduced NKCC1 and Na,K-ATPase expression in murine cochlear lateral wall contribute to conservation of endocochlear potential following a sensorineural hearing loss. Neuroscience Letters. 2011;**488**(2):204-209

[103] Van Eyken E, Van Laer L, Fransen E, Topsakal V, Lemkens N, Laureys W, et al. KCNQ4: A gene for age-related hearing impairment? Human Mutation. 2006;**27**(10):1007-1016

[104] Kubisch C, Schroeder BC, Friedrich T, Lütjohann B, El-Amraoui A, Marlin S, et al. KCNQ4, a novel potassium channel expressed in sensory outer hair cells, is mutated in dominant deafness. Cell. 1999;**96**(3):437-446

[105] Unal M, Tamer L, Doğruer ZN, Yildirim H, Vayisoğlu Y, Camdeviren H. N-acetyltransferase 2 gene polymorphism and presbycusis. The Laryngoscope. 2005;**115**(12):2238-2241

[106] Van Eyken E, Van Camp G, Fransen E, Topsakal V, Hendrickx JJ, Demeester K, et al. Contribution of the N-acetyltransferase 2 polymorphism NAT2*6A to age-related hearing impairment. Journal of Medical Genetics. 2007;**44**(9):570-578

[107] Hein DW. N-acetyltransferase SNPs: Emerging concepts serve as a paradigm for understanding complexities of personalized medicine. Expert Opinion on Drug Metabolism and Toxicology. 2009;**5**(4):353-366

[108] Yan D, Zhu Y, Walsh T, Xie D, Yuan H, Sirmaci A, et al. Mutation of the ATP-gated P2X(2) receptor leads to progressive hearing loss and increased susceptibility to noise. Proceedings of the National Academy of Sciences of the United States of America. 2013;**110**(6):2228-2233

[109] Chen DY, Zhu WD, Chai YC, Chen Y, Sun L, Yang T, et al. Mutation in PCDH15 may modify the phenotypic expression of the 7511T>C mutation in MT-TS1 in a Chinese Han family with maternally inherited nonsyndromic hearing loss. International Journal of Pediatric Otorhinolaryngology. 2015;**79**(10):1654-1657

[110] Zallocchi M, Delimont D, Meehan DT, Cosgrove D. Regulated vesicular trafficking of specific PCDH15 and VLGR1 variants in auditory hair cells. Journal of Neuroscience. 2012;**32**(40):13841-13859

[111] Sakuma N, Moteki H, Azaiez H, Booth KT, Takahashi M, Arai Y, et al. Novel PTPRQ mutations identified in three congenital hearing loss patients with various types of hearing loss. The Annals of Otology, Rhinology, and Laryngology. 2015;**124**(Suppl 1):184S-192S

[112] Ito T, Nishio A, Wangemann P, Griffith AJ. Progressive irreversible hearing loss is caused by stria vascularis degeneration in an Slc26a4-insufficient mouse model of large vestibular aqueduct syndrome. Neuroscience. 2015;**310**:188-197

[113] Girotto G, Morgan A, Krishnamoorthy N, Cocca M, Brumat M, Bassani S, et al. Next generation sequencing and animal models reveal. Frontiers in Genetics. 2019;**10**:142

[114] Morgan A, Vuckovic D, Krishnamoorthy N, Rubinato E, Ambrosetti U, Castorina P, et al. Next-generation sequencing identified SPATC1L as a possible candidate gene for both early-onset and age-related hearing loss. European Journal of Human Genetics. 2019;**27**(1):70-79

[115] Chen J, Ingham N, Kelly J, Jadeja S, Goulding D, Pass J, et al. Spinster homolog 2 (spns2) deficiency causes early onset progressive hearing loss. PLoS Genetics. 2014;**10**(10):e1004688

[116] Lu MH, Takemoto M, Watanabe K, Luo H, Nishimura M, Yano M, et al. Deficiency of sphingomyelin synthase-1 but not sphingomyelin synthase-2 causes hearing impairments in mice. Journal of Physiology. 2012;**590**(16):4029-4044

[117] Di Stazio M, Collesi C, Vozzi D, Liu W, Myers M, Morgan A, et al. TBL1Y: A new gene involved in syndromic hearing loss. European Journal of Human Genetics. 2019;**27**(3):466-474

[118] Ng L, Cordas E, Wu X, Vella KR, Hollenberg AN, Forrest D. Age-related hearing loss and degeneration of cochlear hair cells in mice lacking thyroid hormone receptor β1. Endocrinology. 2015;**156**(10):3853-3865

[119] Ren J, Li H, Lu Y. The determinations of tumor necrosis factor and interleukin 6 in serum of patients with sudden sensorineural hearing loss. Lin Chuang Er Bi Yan Hou Ke Za Zhi. 1998;**12**(7):311-313

[120] Echtay KS. Mitochondrial uncoupling proteins—What is their physiological role? Free Radical Biology and Medicine. 2007;**43**(10):1351-1371

[121] Mattiasson G, Shamloo M, Gido G, Mathi K, Tomasevic G, Yi S, et al. Uncoupling protein-2 prevents neuronal death and diminishes brain dysfunction after stroke and brain trauma. Nature Medicine. 2003;**9**(8):1062-1068

[122] Contrera KJ, Betz J, Deal JA, Choi JS, Ayonayon HN, Harris T, et al. Association of Hearing Impairment and Emotional Vitality in older adults. The Journals of Gerontology. Series B, Psychological Sciences and Social Sciences. 2016;**71**(3):400-404

[123] Kamil RJ, Lin FR. The effects of hearing impairment in older adults on communication partners: A systematic review. Journal of the American Academy of Audiology. 2015;**26**(2):155-182

[124] Christensen VT, Datta Gupta N. Hearing loss and disability exit: Measurement issues and coping strategies. Economics and Human Biology. 2017;**24**:80-91

[125] Moser S, Luxenberger W, Freidl W. The influence of social support and coping on quality of life among elderly with age-related hearing loss. American Journal of Audiology. 2017;**26**(2):170-179

[126] Singh G, Launer S. Social context and hearing aid adoption. Trends in Hearing. 2016;**20**

[127] Hickson L, Meyer C, Lovelock K, Lampert M, Khan A. Factors associated with success with hearing aids in older adults. International Journal of Audiology. 2014;**53**(Suppl 1):S18-S27

[128] Organitzation WH. Multi-country assessment of National Capacity to provide hearing care. Geneva, Switzerland: WHO; 2013. p. 49

[129] Freyer DR, Sung L, Reaman GH. Prevention of hearing loss in children receiving cisplatin chemotherapy. Journal of Clinical Oncology. 2009;**27**(2):317-318. Author reply 8-9

[130] Seidman MD, Khan MJ, Bai U, Shirwany N, Quirk WS. Biologic activity of mitochondrial metabolites on aging and age-related hearing loss. The American Journal of Otology. 2000;**21**(2):161-167

[131] Pouyatos B, Gearhart C, Nelson-Miller A, Fulton S, Fechter LD. Lipoic acid and 6-formylpterin reduce potentiation of noise-induced hearing loss by carbon monoxide: Preliminary investigation. Journal of Rehabilitation Research and Development. 2008;**45**(7):1053-1064

[132] Rybak LP, Whitworth C, Somani S. Application of antioxidants and other agents to prevent cisplatin ototoxicity. The Laryngoscope. 1999;**109**(11):1740-1744

[133] Sha SH, Qiu JH, Schacht J. Aspirin to prevent gentamicin-induced hearing loss. The New England Journal of Medicine. 2006;**354**(17):1856-1857

[134] Van Wijk F, Staecker H, Keithley E, Lefebvre PP. Local perfusion of the tumor necrosis factor alpha blocker infliximab to the inner ear improves autoimmune neurosensory hearing loss. Audiology and Neuro-Otology. 2006;**11**(6):357-365

[135] Wang H, Shi HB, Yin SK. Polyamidoamine dendrimers as gene delivery carriers in the inner ear: How to improve transfection efficiency. Experimental and Therapeutic Medicine. 2011;**2**(5):777-781

[136] Mahmoudian-Sani MR, Mehri-Ghahfarrokhi A, Ahmadinejad F, Hashemzadeh-Chaleshtori M, Saidijam M, Jami MS. MicroRNAs: Effective elements in ear-related diseases and hearing loss. European Archives of Oto-Rhino-Laryngology. 2017;**274**(6):2373-2380

[137] Abbas L, Rivolta MN. The use of animal models to study cell transplantation in neuropathic hearing loss. Hearing Research. 2019;**377**:72-87

[138] Qiu Y, Qiu J. Stem cells: A new Hope for hearing loss therapy. Advances in Experimental Medicine and Biology. 2019;**1130**:165-180

Chapter 8

Overview and Current News in Acute Lymphoblastic Leukemia

Martha Alvarado Ibarra and Jose Antonio De La Peña Celaya

Abstract

The management of acute lymphoblastic leukemia is a challenge in patients of any age range. In the elderly patient, this challenge is further complicated by having to take into account the physical, social, psychological, and emotional factors of this age group, which, together with the complex nature of the disease's biology, give rise to many questions. Although the diagnostic approach of the disease does not differ from that performed in pediatric or young patients, it does in the determination of risk factors and treatment, since many of the determinants of risk have a different value to that assigned in other patients, and, therefore, we cannot apply all available resources in younger patients to facilitate our work. The genetic alterations of ALL are found more frequently in elderly patients, since age is a factor that increases the risk of presenting these alterations. As an example, the prognostic value of the presence of Philadelphia chromosome (t (9:22)) cannot be weighted at the same scale as in pediatric patients. Comorbidities play another important role when it comes to making therapeutic decisions, and there is currently controversy regarding the use of scores designed to determine the physical and physiological status of elderly subjects. Several analyzes have been carried out to define the value and usefulness of these tools in the older patients with ALL; however, work must still be done in this area. The treatment schemes should be adjusted to the needs and specific characteristics of each individual in advanced age. The use of intensive chemotherapy should be discussed within a multidisciplinary team, always considering the benefit of our patients. In the present chapter, the diverse differences in ALL biology will be addressed when compared with those of children and young adults, and with the impact on the different prognostic determinants and their weight at the time of deciding treatment. The need to apply geriatric tools for decision-making and the therapeutic schemes used around the world for elderly people will also be discussed.

Keywords: acute lymphoblastic leukemia, long-term survival, older adults, remission, leukemia-free survival, overall survival, death

1. Introduction

Acute lymphoblastic leukemia (ALL) is a rare disease in the elderly. The prevalence of ALL in patients >60 years of age is reported to be between 16 and 31% of all adult cases. In adults, it represents approximately 20% of all leukemia [1].

The age-adjusted incidence rate of ALL in the United States is 1.58 for every 100,000 persons per year. About 57.2% of the patients diagnosed are under 20 years of age, 26.8% of patients diagnosed are over 45 years of age, and 11% of patients diagnosed are over 65 years of age [2]. The biology of ALL in older patients seems to be significantly different from that in younger patients and may, at least in part, explain the poor treatment outcome. Immunophenotyping and cytogenetic characteristics are among the most important biological differences in comparison with younger adults. The frequency of pre-B-cell ALL and common ALL is higher, and T-cell ALL subtype is under-represented in elderly populations compared with younger patients. The frequency of the Philadelphia chromosome also seems to increase with age and adversely influences complete remission rate and survival. Few reports on the effectiveness and toxicity of therapeutic programs concerning exclusively older patients with ALL have been published so far and only some of them were prospective studies [3].

In some of the studies, age-adapted approaches have been applied in which protocols processed earlier for younger patients have been adopted for older patients. In such modified protocols, chemotherapy was usually less aggressive, especially if it was given for patients with comorbidities and poor performance status. Consequently, in several studies, elderly patients received suboptimal treatment. Death during induction chemotherapy was observed in 7–42% of the patients in particular reports. The overall response rate varied from 12 to 85%. The median overall survival (OS) durations in patients who received a curative approach ranged from 3 to 14 months and from 1 to 14 months in patients treated with palliative therapy. Poor performance status, comorbidities, and high early mortality during intensive chemotherapy are the main reasons for poor treatment results and short OS time. New therapeutic approaches are necessary to improve the outcome in this age group of patients with ALL [4].

The implementation of tools aimed to determining the safety of treatments in elderly patients based on protocols that have previously been applied and validated in younger patients is a common practice today. A recently identified problem when applying these tasks is the underutilization of treatments with curative purposes in this group. An example of this is the CIRS-G scale, widely used to determine the risk of complications in patients with various comorbidities [4]. This phenomenon has been recorded in various efficacies and safety analyzes of treatment for acute lymphoblastic leukemia in elderly patients based on similar scales, where an important survival difference has been observed between the groups treated for curative purposes and those who received reduced therapy. Of course, comorbidities play an important role in these poor results, which forces us to search for new therapeutic options [5].

The clonal origin of ALL has been established using cytogenetic analysis; restriction fragment analysis in female patients, which are heterozygous for polymorphic genes linked to the X chromosome; and analysis of T-cell receptor or immunoglobulin gene rearrangements. The clinical manifestations are very variable and insidious. The symptoms generally reflect bone marrow failure characterized by four syndromes: anemia, hemorrhage, febrile, and infiltrative. Nearly, half of the patients present with some kind of infectious process at diagnosis. Bone infiltration may produce pain and arthralgia. Additionally, close to half the patients have hepatomegaly or splenomegaly [5].

The long-term survival of older adults with acute lymphoblastic leukemia (ALL) who are intensively treated is about 40% [1]. Hematologic remissions are obtained in over 90% of patients, and the depth of these remissions using flow cytometry and molecular techniques is the subject of current studies. It is likely that, with time, new response definitions based on these tests will be established. The adult patients were divided into age 30 years and 30–60 years, because this seemed clinically relevant, and available data best dealt with these age categories.
However, these divisions are not absolute or evidence-based, and an individual's biologic age and general fitness are of paramount importance. There are no randomized studies in older adults that demonstrate "pediatric" approaches to be

superior, and indeed, the single-arm studies are still small scale in this age group, with insufficient follow-up. Much is unknown, but the wide variety of trials being conducted in adults with ALL is heartening [6].

2. Physiopathology

The development of ALL is driven by successive mutations that alter cellular functions promoting

- greater ability for self-renewal,
- greater proliferation,
- blockage of differentiation, and
- resistance to apoptotic signals.

Different hereditary DNA repair disorders can play an important role in the induction of this disease. Furthermore, mutagenic environmental agents, which can be physical (ionizing radiation), chemical (benzene), and biological (HTLV-1), can also be involved. However, in most cases, there are no identifiable etiologic agents. The precise pathogenic events that lead to the development of ALL are unknown. About 5% of the cases are associated with genetic predisposition syndromes. This is the case for children with Down syndrome, who have a 10–30 times greater risk of leukemia and present genetic abnormalities such as hyperdiploidy and t (12; 21) [ETV6-RUNX1], +X, del (9), and alteration in CCAAT//enhacer-binding protein beta (CEBPD). It has been demonstrated that the fusion of P2RY8-CRLF2 and the activation of JAK mutations contribute to 50% of the ALL cases in patients with Down syndrome. Ninety percent have a deletion of IKZF12015. The disorders associated with chromosomal fragility that have been found to predispose to ALL include ataxia-telangiectasia, Nijmegen syndrome, and Bloom syndrome [7]. Patients with ataxia-telangiectasia have 70 times greater risk of leukemia and 250 times greater risk of lymphoma, particularly of T cells. The causal gene, ataxia-telangiectasia mutated (ATM), encodes a protein implicated in DNA repair and regulation of cellular proliferation and apoptosis [2, 7, 8]. Complete genome sequencing studies have identified a number of common allelic variants in four genes (IKZF1, ARID5B, CEBPE, and y CDKN2A) associated with infant ALL. The allelic variant inherited can affect the response to treatment. In utero exposure to X-rays for diagnostic use can confer a slight increase in risk for ALL, which positively correlates with exposure intensity. Data exist that support a causal role for polymorphisms in genes that encode antioxidant enzymes (for example: glutathione S-transferase, nicotinamide adenine dinucleotide phosphate (NADPH), quinone oxidoreductase), folate metabolic enzymes (serine hydroxymethyltransferase and thymidylate synthase), cytochrome 450, methylenetetrahydrofolate reductase, and cell cycle inhibitors [3, 5, 8, 9]. Specific fusion genes have been identified in leukemia, the most noteworthy being KMT2A/AFF1 (also known as MLL-AF4) and ETV6-RUNX1 or TEL-AML1; additionally, there is hyperploid and rearrangements of immunoglobulin or T-cell receptor genes. The acquired genetic anomalies are a hallmark, 80% of all cases contain cytogenetic or molecular lesions with abnormalities in chromosome number (ploidy) and structure. The mechanisms involved include aberrant expression of oncoproteins, loss of tumor suppressor genes, and chromosomal translocations, which generate fusion genes that encode transcription factors of active kinases. A single genetic rearrangement is not enough to induce leukemia. Cooperative mutations are necessary for leukemic transformation and include genetic and epigenetic changes in regulatory growth pathways. Candidate genes identified include deletion of the tumor suppressor locus CDKN2A/CDKN2B and NOTCH1 mutations in T cells. The use of single nucleotide polymorphism (SNP) microarrays suggests that genomic instability is not characteristic of most cases. There is a great variation in the number of alterations in different subtypes of leukemia. The infant cases with rearrangements of the MLL gene had less than one copy number alterations (CNA) per case, suggesting that few genetic lesions are required. Conversely, cases with ETV6-RUNX1 [25] and BCR-ABL1 had more than six CNAs, some containing more than 20 lesions, which support the concept that despite the initiating events that may occur in early infancy, additional lesions are required for the subsequent development of ALL. The lymphoid transcription factor PAX5 encodes a protein involved in evolution and fidelity of the B-cell lineage. The second most frequently affected gene was IKZF1, which encodes the protein IKAROS, required for lymphoid differentiation. IKZF1 is absent in most cases with BCR-ABL1. Approximately, half of the patients expressing BCRABL1 also had deletions in CDKN2A/B and PAX5. This finding suggests that alterations in different signaling pathways are needed to induce leukemia [15]. A special role in this disease is played by the presence of the Philadelphia chromosome t (9; 22), which expresses the BCR-ABL fusion gene, and this has diagnostic, prognostic, and therapeutic implications [3, 6–11].

3. Morphologic diagnosis

The bone marrow aspiration test is fundamental to confirm the presence of lymphoblasts (by morphology and/or cytochemistry with special stains that include a negative MPO in 100% of cells, Periodic Acid-Shiff (PAS) (+) in 70–80%, and acid phosphatase (+) in the case of T lymphoblast). The WHO suggests greater than 20% as diagnosis criteria (if the percentage is lower, one must search for extramedullary disease at the nodal level to differentiate from the diagnosis of lymphoblastic lymphoma). The bone marrow aspiration is hypercellular 95–100% of the time; however, in those cases where the aspirate is "dry" (packed bone marrow), which corresponds to 1–2% of the cases, a bone biopsy must be carried out for histopathological confirmation. Based on morphology, the French-American-British (FAB) classification identifies three types of ALL [7, 8, 12].

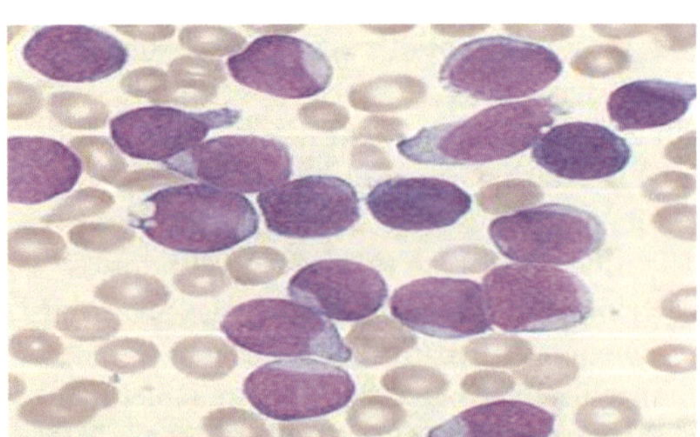

The first step to integrate the diagnosis of ALL is the morphological identification of lymphoblasts. For this, it is necessary to perform a bone marrow aspirate and be observed directly under a microscope by an expert in hematology, which can be supported in other tests like special stains, as in the case of myeloperoxidase, which must be negative in all the malignant cells observed; PAS staining, which is considered positive for ALL when observed in 70–80% of cells with malignant morphology and acid phosphatase, which is used for T-cell differentiation. Regarding manual cell counting, it is necessary that the presence of 20% or more cells with malignant characteristics, as indicated by the criteria of the WHO classification, in case this criterion is not met, can be replaced by others such as the documentation of extramedullary disease. It is important to specify that most of the times, we may have difficulties in trying to obtain the sample for the bone marrow aspirate, since the large number of cells within the medullary space condition the presence of the phenomenon of "dry" aspiration; in these cases, we must carry out bone biopsy in a mandatory manner.

3.1 Images ALL

The French-American-British (FAB) classification that was used commonly earlier includes:

- L1—around 25–30% of adult cases and 85% of childhood cases of ALL are of this subtype. In this type, small cells are seen with:
    - regular nuclear shape
    - homogeneous chromatin
    - small or absent nucleolus
    - scanty cytoplasm
- L2—around 70% of adult cases and 14% of childhood cases are of this type. The cells are large and/or have varied shapes with:
    - irregular nuclear shape
    - heterogeneous chromatin
    - large nucleolus
- L3—this is a rarer subtype with only 1–2% cases. In this type, the cells are large and uniform with vacuoles (bubble-like features) in the cytoplasm overlying the nucleus.

In an initial effort, the French-American-British (FAB) was given the task of subclassifying this type of leukemia according to various morphological characteristics in order to try to determine the behavior and prognosis of each type based on its morphology; this is how the FAB morphological classification was born, which subdivides the ALL into three types:

- L1: this subtype is characterized by presenting cells with a regular nucleus, homogeneous chromatin, small or absent nucleoli, and scarce cytoplasm. It represents the majority of the ALL in children observed in up to 85%, while in adults, it is seen between 30% and 70% of the times.
- L2: unlike the previous one, this subclassification is seen mostly in adults (70%) and its morphology is opposite to L1: chromatin is heterogeneous, the nucleus irregular, and with multiple nucleoli.

- L3: the least frequent of the three, is reported between 1 and 2% of the time. Its main characteristic is the large number of vacuoles (bubbles) that these cells present in their cytoplasm. The shape of the nucleus may vary.

3.2 Revised version of FAB

WHO proposed a classification of ALL that was to be the revised version of the FAB classification.

This used the immunophenotypic classification that includes:

- Acute lymphoblastic leukemia/lymphoma or formerly L1 and L2 this has subtypes including:
    - precursor B acute lymphoblastic leukemia/lymphoma: this has genetic subtypes including t(12,21)(p12,q22) TEL/AML-1, t(1,19)(q23;p13) PBX/E2A, t(9,22)(q34;q11) ABL/BCR and T(V,11)(V;q23) V/MLL
    - precursor T acute lymphoblastic leukemia/lymphoma
- Burkitt's leukemia/lymphoma or formerly L3
- biphenotypic acute leukemia

The WHO performed a new categorization of acute lymphoblastic leukemia, based on cytogenetic alterations present in this disease. This classification considered what was previously described in the FAB classification being possible to make an indirect correlation between the morphological findings and the alterations listed in the categories of the WHO classification. In this way, those leukemias that are traditionally classified in the FAB groups L1 and L2 can belong to the group of leukemia of precursors B with alterations such as: t (12; 21) (p12, q22) TEL/AML-1, t (1; 19) (q23; p13) PBX/E2A, t (9; 22) (q34; q11) ABL/BCR, and T (V, 11) (V; q23) V/MLL. Those traditionally classified as FAB L3 correlate with Burkitt's leukemia/lymphoma; T-cell leukemias are still an independent group and are considered another group where those that meet criteria for two different lineages are included.

4. Lineage

The proportion of B-lineage ALL is higher in patients older (75–89%) than 60 years compared to patients younger (59–66%) than 60 years. Accordingly the incidence of T-ALL is lower in older (8–12%) compared to younger (29%) patients [5–7]. A population-based study showed that cytogenetics were less frequently attempted in older (73%) compared with younger (85–91%) patients. The proportion of patients with Philadelphia chromosome positive (Ph+) t(9;22), t(8;14), t(14;18), or complex aberrations increased with age [11]; Ph+ ALL accounted for 24–36% in older patients vs. 15–19% in younger patients. Considering the consequences resulting from diagnostic characterization, it should be self-evident that complete diagnostic characterization is required in all patients with ALL, regardless of age [13, 14].

There are several important differences in the biology of lymphoblastic leukemia in patients over 60 years compared to those under this age, although we know that B-lineage leukemia is the most common in adults, the frequency between both groups can vary reporting a little more frequent in those over 60 years (75–89%/59–66%), another more radical difference is the presentation of leukemia of T lineage, which is more common in adults under 60 years (29%) than in elderly patients (12%) [5–7]. Cytogenetic alterations of importance for the prognosis, such as Philadelphia chromosome (Ph+) t (9; 22), t (8; 14), t (14; 18), or complex karyotype are observed more frequently as the patient's age increases [11]. Although the search for cytogenetic alterations is crucial to define the risk and possible response to treatment of acute leukemia, this analysis is not carried out in most elderly patients (73%), contrary to the young patients, who have available cytogenetic studies in up to 91%. The importance of this difference lies in the fact, already mentioned, of the increase in the frequency of high-risk alterations, as an example Ph+ ALL can be found in up to 36% of cases, which have different therapeutic approaches to those that do not suffer from this alteration [13, 14].

As in other B-cell malignancies, monoclonal antibodies to CD20 or CD228 are being tested as adjuncts to chemotherapy in the hope that they will increase remission depth and improve survival without increasing hematologic toxicity. About 60–80% of B-cell ALL patients express these antigens at variable densities, but there is little evidence linking antigen expression to response. CD20 expression may be associated with a worse prognosis, so it is logical to investigate CD20 antibodies in randomized trials, and it may improve the outcome [15, 16].

4.1 Immunophenotyping

Blasts in pre-B ALL can be initially identified using an SSC vs. a CD45 plot. These blasts have low SSC (many times smaller than normal lymphocytes) and dim to negative CD45.

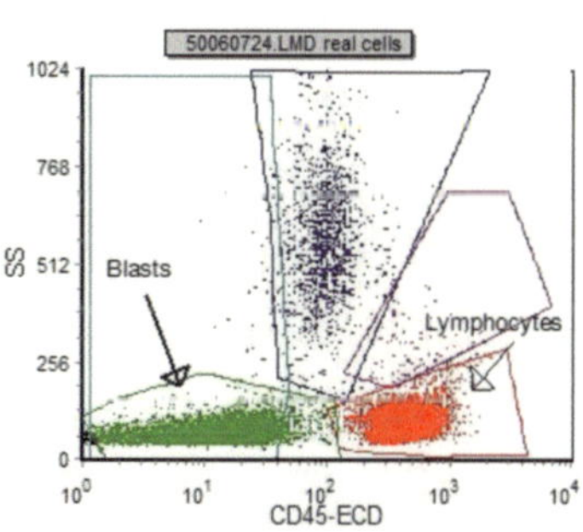

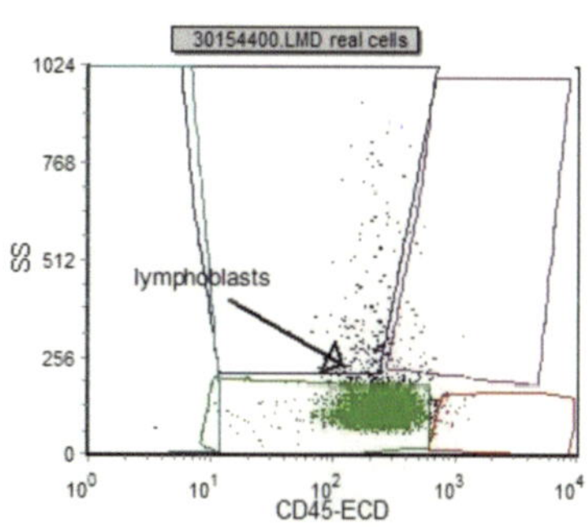

Example peripheral blood with CD45 negative B lymphoblasts and characteristically small (low SSC)

Example bone marrow with CD45 dim B lymphoblasts.

Once the blasts are identified and gated, the following markers are useful in the classification of pre-B ALL:

Marker	Prevalence
CD10	89%
CD13	5%
CD19	100%
CD20	24%
CD22	69%
CD33	31%
CD34	76%

Marker	Prevalence
CD45 (bright)	2%
CD45 (moderate)	33%
CD45 (dim)	36%
CD45 (negative)	29%
CD56	36%
CD79a	88%
CD117	0%
Cytoplasmic IgM	22%
HLA Dr	98%
TdT	91%

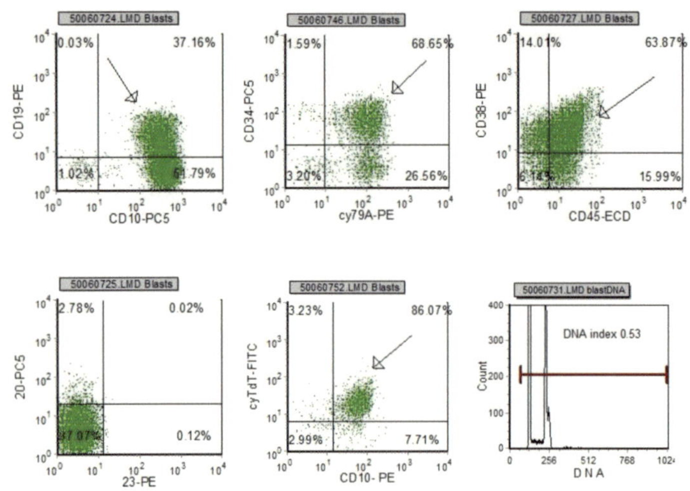

Pre B ALL cells characteristically coexpress CD10 and CD19. In addition, CD20 and CD23 (other B cell

Expression of CD34 and TdT indicates immaturity and is characteristic in pre B ALL. Cytoplasmic expression of CD79 confirms B cell lineage.

CD38 is an expression of immaturity. The ploidy as seen by the DNA Histogram, indicates a hypodiploidy (DI=0.53)

Included are marking prevalences.

The phenotype of the blasts is an independent prognostic parameter. B-ALL is subdivided into following:

- *Early Pre-B ALL*: TdT+, CD19+, CD10-
- *Common ALL*: CD19+, CD10+/CALLA+
- *Pre-B ALL*: CD10+/–, CD19+, HLA DR+, cytoplasmic IgM+
- *Mature B ALL*: CD10+, CD19+, CD20+, CD22+, surface IgM+

4.2 Immunophenotype of T-lineage ALL

T-cell ALL constitutes approximately 25% of all adult cases of ALL. T-cell markers are CD1a, CD2, CD3 (membrane and cytoplasm), CD4, CD5, CD7, and CD8.

CD2, CD5, and CD7 antigens are markers of the most immature T cells , but none of them is absolutely lineage-specific, so that the unequivocal diagnosis of T-ALL rests on the demonstration of surface/cytoplasmic CD3. In T-ALL, the expression of CD10 is quite common (25%) and not specific; CD34 and myeloid antigens CD13 and/or CD33 can be expressed too. Recognized T-ALL subsets are the following: pro-T EGIL T-I (cCD3+, CD7+), pre-T EGIL T-II (cCD3+, CD7+, and CD5/CD2+), cortical T EGIL T-III (cCD3+, CD1a+, and sCD3+/−), and mature-T EGIL T-IV (cCD3+, sCD3+, and CD1a−). Finally, a novel subgroup that was recently characterized is represented by the so-called ETP-ALL (early-T precursor), which shows characteristic immunophenotypic features, namely lack of CD1a and CD8 expression, weak CD5 expression, and expression of at least one myeloid and/or stem cell marker [17].

4.3 Mixed phenotype acute leukemia

With currently refined diagnostic techniques, the occurrence of acute leukemia of ambiguous cell lineage, i.e., mixed phenotype acute leukemia (MPAL) is relatively rare (<4%) [19]. These cases express one of the following feature: (1) coexistence of two separate blast cell populations (i.e., T- or B-cell ALL plus either myeloid or monocytic blast cells), (2) single leukemic population of blast cells co-expressing B- or T-cell antigens and myeloid antigens, and (3) same plus expression of monocytic antigens. For myelo-monocytic lineage, useful diagnostic antigens are MPO or nonspecific esterase, CD11c, CD14, CD64 and lysozyme; for B-lineage, CD19 plus CD79a, cytoplasmic CD22 and CD10 (one or two of the latter according to staining intensity of CD19); and for T-lineage, cytoplasmic or surface CD3. Recognized entities include Ph+ MPAL (B/myeloid or rarely T/myeloid), t(v;11q23); MLL rearranged MPAL, and genetically uncharacterized B or T/myeloid MPAL. Very rare cases express trilineage involvement (B/T/myeloid). Lack of lineage-specific antigens (MPO, cCD3, cCD22) is observed in the ultrarare acute undifferentiated leukemia. In a recent review of 100 such cases, 59% were B/myeloid, 35% T/myeloid, 4% B/T lymphoid, and 2% B/T/myeloid. Outcome was overall better following ALL rather than AML therapy [7, 16, 18, 19].

4.4 NK cell ALL

CD56, a marker of natural killer (NK) cell differentiation, defines a rare subgroup of about 3% of adult ALL cases, which often display other early T-cell antigens, CD7 CD2 CD5, and sometimes cCD3. True NK ALL is very rare (TdT+, CD56+, other T markers negative, and un-rearranged TCR genes). This diagnosis rely on the demonstration of early NK-specific CD94 or CD161 antigens [18, 19].

4.5 Diagnostic cytogenetics

Cytogenetics represents an important step in ALL classification. Conventional karyotyping can be helpful in the identification of recurrent translocations, as well as gain and loss of gross chromosomal material; however, the major limitation of this technique is that in some cases, leukemic cells fail to enter metaphase. However, fluorescence in situ hybridization (FISH) can enable the detection and direct visualization of virtually all investigated chromosomal abnormalities in ALL, with a sensitivity of around 99%. Finally, array-comparative genomic hybridization (array-CGH, a-CGH) and single nucleotide polymorphisms (SNP) arrays can permit the identification of cryptic and/or submicroscopic changes in the genome. Karyotype changes found in ALL include both numerical and structural alterations, which have profound prognostic significance. With these premises in mind, the karyotype changes that occur in ALL can be roughly subdivided in those associated, respectively, with a relatively good, intermediate, and poor prognosis. However, it must be kept in mind that the incidence of certain aberrations is very low, and that for some of them, the prognostic impact can be strongly affected by the type and intensiveness of therapy administered [8, 20].

5. Clinical status

Features associated with large tumor mass or rapid progression, such as high white blood cell count, mediastinal tumors, or other organ involvement, appear to be less common in older patients. Even "smoldering" ALL is observed in some cases. Most studies report a lower proportion of males among older ALL patients. Secondary ALL after myelodysplastic syndromes or other malignant disease may become increasingly important, particularly in older patients; so far, very limited data are available. Performance status often deteriorates in older patients with onset of disease. In two studies, 30–43% of patients older than age 60 years vs. 18–22% of younger patients had a performance status of 2 or more. Therefore, it is important not only to consider the current general condition in newly admitted older ALL patients but also to discern their status before the onset of leukemia-associated symptoms [17, 21].

The determination of the clinical status at the moment of making the diagnosis provides us with information about the global state of the patient, so that we can make better decisions. This varies in comparison with the younger groups in questions such as the low initial presentation of large tumor mass, identified by the elevated white blood cells count in the peripheral blood, the rare extranodal affection and even in some cases being observed, apparently "benign" clinical presentation with low tumor burden. A smaller proportion of male patients in this group have also been observed as compared with younger groups. Secondary leukemia, which we define as that which occurs after a premalignant pathology, most frequently myelodysplastic syndrome, or after treatment of nonhematological neoplasms, is a condition that has been observed more and more frequently in recent years. However, there is little data to help us determine its nature. It is important to assess these patients comprehensively in order to determine their physical and health status prior to the onset of symptoms related to leukemia [17, 21].

6. Comorbidity

Of older ALL patients, 60–70% suffer from comorbidities, but most studies did not refer to validated scoring systems. The German multicentre study group for adult ALL (GMALL) identified comorbidities according to the Charlson score in 84% of the patients older than 55 years, with diabetes (46%), vascular disease (18%), heart failure (15%), and chronic lung disease (12%) being the most frequent. In addition, renal insufficiency, anemia, osteoporosis, dementia, and depression are probably the most relevant comorbidities for potential adjustment of treatment. About 8–16% had a history of prior malignant disease. I recommend a systematic evaluation and documentation of comorbidities based on a checklist or a score, since this is essential for planning an optimal treatment strategy [4, 5, 18, 23].

Comorbidities in elderly patients with ALL require a specialized and detailed approach. The German multicentre study group for adult ALL (GMALL) recommends the use of the Charlson scale for the determination of risk due to comorbidities; this assessment must be done in an integral manner, together with the physics, biochemistry, and cytomolecular evaluation of the disease [4]. Multiple systemic diseases can afflict elderly patients with ALL: diabetes, hypertension, heart failure, and renal failure are some of the most frequently reported in the various studies conducted. Age-specific conditions such as dementia or osteoporosis that can negatively impact the patient's performance before and after treatment should not be left aside. It is also important to evaluate, monitor and, if necessary, treat alterations in the emotional state of the elderly patient, since depression and anxiety are not infrequent conditions in this group [5, 18, 22].

7. Prognostic factors in older ALL patients

Now, we have a better understanding of the factors that determine survival, but these will require reexamination as we introduce novel therapies. Cytogenetic findings such as Philadelphia chromosome positivity, t (4; 11), complex cytogenetic abnormalities (more than five chromosomal changes), and low hypodiploidy/near triploidy result in inferior survival. Some of these changes are more common in older adults. Other conventional factors such as increasing age, high white blood cell count, and B-cell disease (rather than T-cell disease) still hold true and predict higher failure rates with standard chemotherapy. However, many of these factors are also associated with a higher relapse rate after allografting, and it is not necessarily the case that bone marrow transplantation (BMT) is the solution for patients with adverse prognostic features. Combining these factors may allow individualization of therapy, a prospect not previously possible in this rare condition. As well as undertreating patients with ALL with chemotherapy that is likely to fail, prognostic factors should be used to avoid over treating better prognosis patients with allogeneic transplants that have a high upfront risk and may result in chronic graft-versus host disease (GVHD), infertility, and secondary malignancy. Chemotherapy and transplant have complementary roles in ALL management, and a pragmatic approach is required to deliver the best outcomes. The role of BMT is likely to increase, especially with the promising results of reduced-intensity allografting, but conversely, the use of BMT should be reduced if advances in nontransplant therapy improve cure rates [11, 17, 20, 23].

Increasing age itself is one of the most relevant prognostic factors for outcome of ALL from childhood to old age. Since older patients show opposite problems, namely higher mortality and relapse rates, prognostic factors for both have to be analyzed. Prognostic factors for relapse risk in younger ALL patients are probably also valid in older patients, such as early and mature T-ALL, pro-B ALL, elevated white blood cell count, and Ph+ ALL; however, their predictive value is somewhat diluted by mortality risks. Evaluation of minimal residual disease (MRD) has demonstrated that persistence of MRD is associated with a relapse rate above 90% in younger patients despite continued intensive chemotherapy. Few data on the prognostic impact of MRD are available in older patients. In one study, only 11% of the older patients with molecular failure after first consolidation remained in complete response (CR) compared with 68% of those with molecular remission. In older patients with less intensive therapy, a higher rate of MRD persistence and an even poorer outcome can be expected. Therefore, prospective evaluation of MRD in older patients is essential to identify those who could benefit from alternative experimental treatments, if they were available [18–20, 24].

Some poor prognosis factor applicable to young patients can also be in elderly patients, which tells us of the profound impact they have on the biology of the disease: the T lineage and the positive Phi chromosome are a pair of these. The persistence of positive minimal residual disease is directly related to an increased frequency of relapse after remission; it is estimated that young patients with positive MRD will relapse up to 90% despite receiving intensive CT. We do not have such exact estimates of how much the likelihood of relapse increases when this phenomenon occurs in older patients, but it has been estimated in some studies that only 11% of these who presented with MRD positive remain in response to the disease. Prospective studies that answer these questions are required; however, it is necessary to determine MRD in elderly patients as part of the management and surveillance protocols [18–20, 23].

In the GMALL study for older patients, we identified comorbidity score, age, and performance status before onset of leukemia as prognostic factors with significant impact on early mortality. Interestingly, Eastern Cooperative Oncology Group (ECOG) status of 2 or more was documented in 7% of the patients before onset of leukemia-associated symptoms, but in 38% after onset. The strong correlation of performance status with mortality was confirmed by others.

For assessing prognosis in an older ALL patient, it is essential to identify features suitable for predicting high risk of early mortality resulting from complications. These features can help determine whether a patient has any chance of benefiting from intensive treatment. For this purpose, I would consider performance status before onset of leukemia, comorbidities, and geriatric assessment and would not rely on scores, which are calculated on the basis of historical patient cohorts.

In addition, prognostic factors for response to antileukemic treatment and relapse risk must be considered. Because of the lack of confirmed prognostic factors for older ALL patients, my approach would be to take known prognostic factors for younger patients into consideration, but to focus on MRD evaluation as an individual prognostic feature that can cover the impact of biologic factors and also treatment intensity, compliance, and other unknown features [21, 26].

In the case of patients with characteristics that could increase the risk of early mortality when starting treatment, we must be careful in how to approach this last parameter. Several groups dedicated to the analysis of prognostic factors in special groups of patients have determined a series of variants and elements that could guide the clinic when defining the risk of death of his patient. The GMALL group determined, in a prospective analysis, that the low physical status (ECOG status of 2 or more) prior to the onset of leukemia symptoms correlates with earlier mortality and in those patients who already have a diagnosis, this score is seen duplicated at the beginning of the symptomatology. To be able to carry out a complete evaluation of elderly patients, it is necessary to apply tools that are useful in most clinical scenarios and that confer a high degree of reliability with respect to their predictive power of prognosis. It is therefore necessary to apply validated geriatric scores and specific scores of the patient for known morbidities in order to achieve the most complete vision possible before the diagnosis, in order to guide the treatment and its intensity [21].

In addition to this, we must define what prognostic factors for relapse should be applied to these patients after treatment is initiated. Although several of them already known with importance in young group can also be applied to elderly patients, it should be determined which are more specific for this last group [26].

7.1 Philadelphia ALL

One-quarter of all adults have Philadelphia chromosome, and the incidence increases with age. Until the results of recent studies in older patients became available, most patients with Philadelphia ALL were managed with intensive chemotherapy and a tyrosine kinase inhibitor (TKI). Imatinib has improved the CR rate in a number of trials to 90% and makes more patients eligible for transplant. Imatinib-resistant mutations are increasingly reported, and these should be sought in relapsed and refractory patients. Dasatinib, which inhibits tyrosine and src kinases, holds considerable promise. It may also be effective in CNS disease. There are no randomized comparisons with imatinib, although it is a more potent inhibitor of tyrosine kinase in vitro. Recent studies from Italy and France with dasatinib alone in older patients have achieved very high remission rates with encouraging short-term survival. Good minimal residual disease (MRD) responses correlated with outcome. Data regarding the combination of dasatinib and intensive chemotherapy are lacking. It is possible that less conventional induction therapy may be required and that allogeneic stem cell transplantation (SCT) may not be mandatory. The remarkable effectiveness of TKI therapy, in some studies without chemotherapy or allografting, has made us consider de-escalation of therapy, but the long-term results of these less intensive approaches are unknown, and allografting is the only known cure. The effect of pretransplant MRD status on outcome is unclear [27, 28].

A study of 267 patients (prior to the TKI era) showed allogeneic transplant to be superior to chemotherapy, with 44 and 36% surviving 5 years after sibling and unrelated donor SCT, respectively. However, only 28% of patients proceeded to a CR1 allograft, reducing its impact, and making it important that we improve no transplant therapy (and improve access to transplant). The Minneapolis group reported 50% survival in 14 patients who received reduced-intensity conditioning (RIC) allografts from cord or sibling donors. TKIs were used only for morphologic or molecular relapse posttransplant. Studies of TKI posttransplant that examine dose, duration, and molecular response are urgently required; this is the subject of studies from the German and UK groups that are soon to be reported [28, 29].

7.2 Therapy

The goal of remission induction therapy is to achieve remission without undue toxicity with a hematologic recovery that permits further therapy to be promptly given. Most regimens use prednisolone or dexamethasone, vincristine, daunorubicin, and asparaginase, with later exposure to cyclophosphamide and Ara-C (cytosine arabinoside or cytarabine). Hyper-cyclophosphamide, vincristine, doxorubicin, and dexamethasone (CVAD), which does not contain L-asparaginase, achieves high complete remission (CR) rates in newly diagnosed patients and is a reasonable alternative for induction therapy, but has not been shown to be superior to more traditional induction protocols. Dexamethasone is preferred to prednisolone because of superior lymphocytotoxicity, better central nervous system (CNS) penetration, and fewer thromboembolic events; these data are derived from pediatric studies. Poly(ethylene glycol)-asparaginase may be associated with more effective asparagine depletion, and this in turn may lead to better outcomes. But this requires a randomized comparison. The safety and optimum dose of this drug require further study in adults [25, 26, 30].

Population-based study registries give an impression on the overall outcome of unselected older ALL patients. Survival rates in patients aged 60 years were 12% at 5 years in Northern England. For those aged between 65 and 74 years, survival was 25% in Sweden where outcome further decreased to 10% in patients aged 74 years. Five-year OS in patients aged 60–69 years increased from 8% in the years 1992–2001 to 20% in the years 2002–2011, whereas only marginal improvements from 5 to 10% were observed for patients aged 70 years. Palliative treatment: some 30–70% of the older patients are allocated to palliative therapy mainly due to poor performance status at diagnosis. Most studies have shown an advantage of more intensive therapy such as higher CR rate, lower early death, better remission duration, and median survival compared with palliative treatment according to protocols for adult ALL patients. The majority of published data are based on results reported for the subgroup of older patients treated within protocols designed for adult ALL in general. One large data set confirmed considerable mortality of 18%. The conclusion that induction therapy designed for younger patients may be too intensive for older patients. Patients may acquire severe infections, nonpredefined treatment modifications occur frequently, and treatments may be interrupted or even stopped due to severe complications. Overall, potential conclusions from these studies are very limited. Prospective studies of protocols for older ALL patients specifically designed for older ALL patients have the theoretical aim to provide a chance of cure on the one hand and to limit toxicity, early mortality, and hospitalization duration on the other hand, and the therapy maintains as much quality of life as possible. One central question is whether and/or which anthracycline has to be included in induction regimens for older patients, because these drugs contribute considerably to bone marrow toxicity [5, 6, 15, 31]. One approach is the use of idarubicin in induction, based on a potentially lower cardiac and hepatic toxicity. The results of liposomal anthracyclines in elderly ALL are not convincing so far. Asparaginase is an essential compound in the treatment of ALL. The PETHEMA group reported the results of an intensive induction regimen, including asparaginase for older ALL patients. The early death rate, mainly due to infection, was rather high (36%) and was reduced after omission of asparaginase and cyclophosphamide. A high early mortality rate (29%) and a number of complications including infections (71%), cardiac toxicity (18%), and hyperglycemia (24%) were also observed in another trial utilizing asparaginase during induction therapy. Furthermore, a pediatric-based regimen using pegylated asparaginase during induction in older patients revealed grade 3–4 bilirubin increases in 33% of the patients. Thrombosis and pancreatitis are other relevant toxicities of asparaginase. Altogether, there is some evidence that the use of asparaginase during induction therapy may be associated with increased risks in older patients. Therefore, it would be advisable to start asparaginase in older patients later during consolidation. The majority of complications in older ALL patients is observed during induction; thus, there is still space for intensification of consolidation therapy [14, 23, 32]. Based on this assumption, a consensus treatment protocol for older patients with ALL was defined by the European Working Group for Adult ALL (EWALL). The 4-week, pediatric-based induction comprises dexamethasone, vincristine, and idarubicin in phase 1 and cyclophosphamide and cytarabine in phase 2. Consolidation consists of six alternating cycles with intermediate-dose methotrexate combined with asparaginase and high-dose cytarabine, followed by maintenance. The median age at enrollment was 66 (56–73) years with 22% at 70 years. The incidence of grade 3–4 cytopenias was 90%, and infections during phases 1 and 2 of induction occurred in 16 and 25% of the patients, respectively. Toxicities were less pronounced during consolidation, and asparaginase was well tolerated. CR, survival, and continuous CR rates after 1 year were 85, 61, and 49%, respectively. Another report based on the same backbone showed CR rates of 74% and an OS of 30% at 2 years [18, 20, 33]. The authors also observed grade 3–4 infections in 62% of the patients during induction therapy with a median duration of neutropenia of 24 days, whereas consolidation was far better tolerated even when including the use of asparaginase [18, 20, 23, 34]. The GMALL has conducted thus far the largest prospective trial specifically designed for older patients with Ph/BCR–ABL-negative ALL. Pediatric (Berlin-Frankfurt Munster)-based, dose-reduced induction therapy with idarubicin, dexamethasone, vincristine, cyclophosphamide, and cytarabine was followed by alternating consolidation cycles for 1 year and maintenance. Patients with CD201 ALL received rituximab in combination with chemotherapy. The median age of this cohort was 67 (55–85) years. In 268 patients, the CR rate was 76%, early death rate 14%, mortality in CR 6%, continuous remission 32%, and survival 23% at 5 years. Patients aged 75 years with an Eastern Cooperative Oncology Group performance status below 2 had an 86% CR rate, 10% early death, and 36% survival at 3 years. Interestingly, the replacement of triple intrathecal therapy during induction resulted in a reduced early mortality. Moderate intensification of consolidation as in the EWALL regimen, with inclusion of high-dose cytarabine and intermediate-dose methotrexate and native *Escherichia coli* asparaginase was tolerated [24, 26, 30].

Overall, mortality in CR was 6% only. Overall, pediatric-based regimens in ALL are undoubtedly successful and should be scheduled with prospectively defined adaptations with respect to tolerability in older patients. The most important modification of induction therapy in older patients is probably the omission of asparaginase, and the flexible, reduced dose of anthracyclines. In consolidation, intensified treatment should be attempted, and during this treatment phase, even asparaginase may be surprisingly well tolerated at moderate doses [29, 34]. In this treatment, patients aged 55–70 years and 70–75 years tolerated pegylated asparaginase at dose levels of 1000 and 500 U/m^2, respectively, as single-drug interim therapy during consolidation. Combination with high-dose methotrexate will be further explored and careful use is recommended in patients with preexisting liver disease. [23, 24, 26, 30, 35]. Nowadays, older patients with Ph+ ALL may have a better chance to achieve a CR than patients with Ph+ ALL. The use of TKIs upfront is most promising. The GMALL conducted a first randomized study to evaluate the efficacy of imatinib single-drug induction compared with chemotherapy. The remission rates were 96 and 50%, respectively. Only 11% of the patients achieved a molecular remission. A follow-up including nonrandomized data yielded a CR rate of 88% in 121 patients, together with a 22% 5-year survival rate. The Gruppo Italiano Malattie Ematologiche dell'Adulto trial used imatinib (800 mg) with prednisone for induction, followed by imatinib single-drug treatment. The CR rate, survival, and disease-free survival were 100, 74, and 48%, respectively, after 1 year. A subsequent trial with dasatinib (140 mg) and prednisone, followed by dasatinib single-drug treatment, was not specifically designed for older patients (range, 24–76 years). The CR rate was 92% and survival was 69% at 20 months. Postremission therapy was at the discretion of the treating physician and 14 of 19 patients with TKI monotherapy relapsed with a high frequency of T315I mutations [31, 33, 35]. Another trial was based on a rotating schedule with 6 weeks of nilotinib treatment alternating with imatinib treatment. In 39 patients, the CR rate was 94% and the OS at 1 year was 79%. Nearly, all relapsed patients in this trial showed mutations associated with TKI resistance. The largest prospective study so far in older patients with Ph+ ALL used an EWALL chemotherapy backbone with vincristine, dexamethasone, and dasatinib (140 mg) for induction. Consolidation and maintenance according to the EWALL backbone was combined with intermittent dasatinib applications. In 71 patients, the CR rate was 96%. The regimen was feasible and the survival after 5 years of follow-up was 36%, which is promising. Persistent MRD above 0.1% after induction and consolidation was associated with poorer remission duration of only 5 months. A subsequent EWALL trial with a similar backbone but with nilotinib (400 mg twice daily) instead of dasatinib was started subsequently. Again, a high CR rate of 97% was reported. About 30% of patients achieved a complete molecular remission after induction. Overall, there is increasing evidence that second-generation TKIs in combination with dose-reduced chemotherapy can induce very high CR rates with low mortality in older patients. The rate of molecular remissions appears to be higher compared with imatinib-based regimens. Moderate intensive consolidation therapies in combination with TKIs are tolerated well. Long-term results have to be assessed after 5 or more years and show a still high rate of relapses. New approaches may include reduced intensity stem cell transplantation (SCT), MRD-based change of TKIs, or use of new immunotherapies [23, 36, 37].

In other study, 127 patients with ALL were enrolled including 26 elderly patients (≥60 years) and 101 younger adult patients (<60 years). The median follow-up durations were 6.0 months (range, 0.4–113.2) in the elderly patients and 21.7 months (range, 1.0–122.7) in the younger patients. The median age of the younger patients with ALL was 30 years (range, 15–58), whereas that of the elderly patients with ALL was 65 years (range, 60–82). No significant differences in the baseline characteristics of the two groups were observed, except in history of malignancy; a larger portion of elderly patients with ALL had a history of malignancy ($p = 0.001$). The composition of ALL subtypes and the frequencies of Ph+ status were not statistically significant between the two groups. The peripheral blood sample laboratory findings showed more severe anemia in younger adult patients with ALL than in the elderly patients ($p = 0.023$); of 26 elderly patients with ALL, abnormal karyotypes were found in 14 patients (53.8%) [38, 39].

All patients, with the exception of two elderly patients who received supportive care only, received induction chemotherapy. About half of the elderly patients (12 patients, 46.2%) received the VPDL regimen as an induction therapy. Five elderly patients (19.2%) were administered the VPD regimen, and one (3.8%) was administered the hyper-CVAD (cyclophosphamide 300 mg/m^2, D1–3; vincristine 2 mg D4,11; Adriamycin 50 mg/m^2, D4; dexamethasone 40 mg D1–4, D11–14) regimen. The overall CR rate was much higher in the younger adult patients than that in the elderly patients (94.1 vs. 57.7%, $p < 0.001$). Early mortality within 3 months from the start of induction chemotherapy was remarkably higher in the elderly patients (26.9% vs. 5.0%, $p = 0.003$).

The median number of postremission consolidation therapy sessions was three (range, 1–5) in the elderly patients with ALL. The regimen in the elderly patients was vincristine and prednisolone in seven patients. Two patients received only imatinib due to severe comorbidities. One patient received the CALGB 9251 regimen, and the other patient received nonmyeloablative hematopoietic stem cell transplantation (HSCT) from a matched sibling donor. Of 15 elderly patients who achieved CR, only 11 received postremission therapy. The overall nondisease-related mortality rate in the elderly patients was higher than that in the younger adult patients.

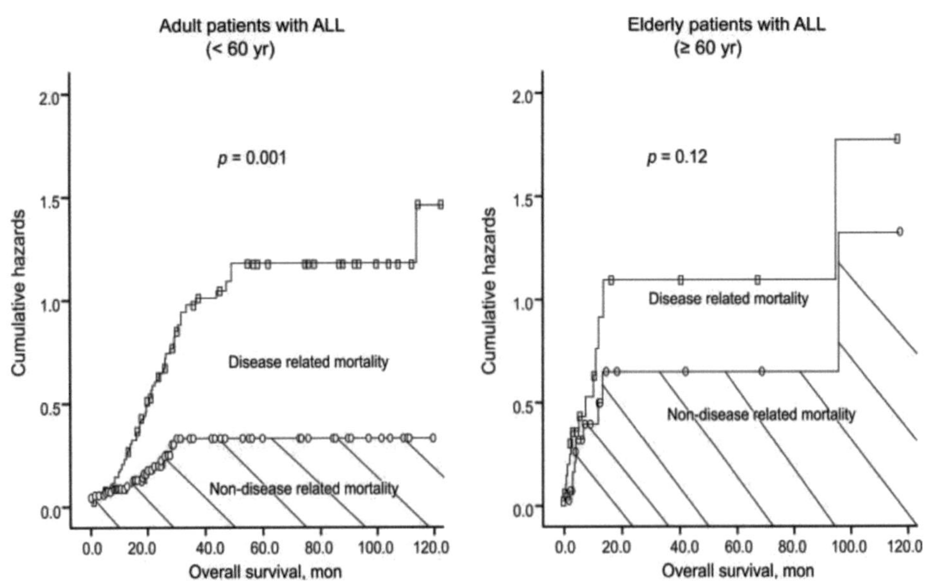

Cumulative hazards of disease-related and nondisease-related mortality in younger adult patients (<60 years) with acute lymphoblastic leukemia (ALL) and in elderly patients (≥60 years) with ALL ($p = 0.001$ and 0.12, respectively).

The median OS of the younger patients was 26.3 months (95% confidence interval [CI], 19.6–33.0), whereas that of the elderly patients was 10.3 months (95% CI, 3.5–17.2) ($p = 0.003$). The survival difference according to age was not reproduced in the subpopulation of patients with Ph-positive ALL (data not shown), but was consistently found in the patients with Ph-negative ALL.

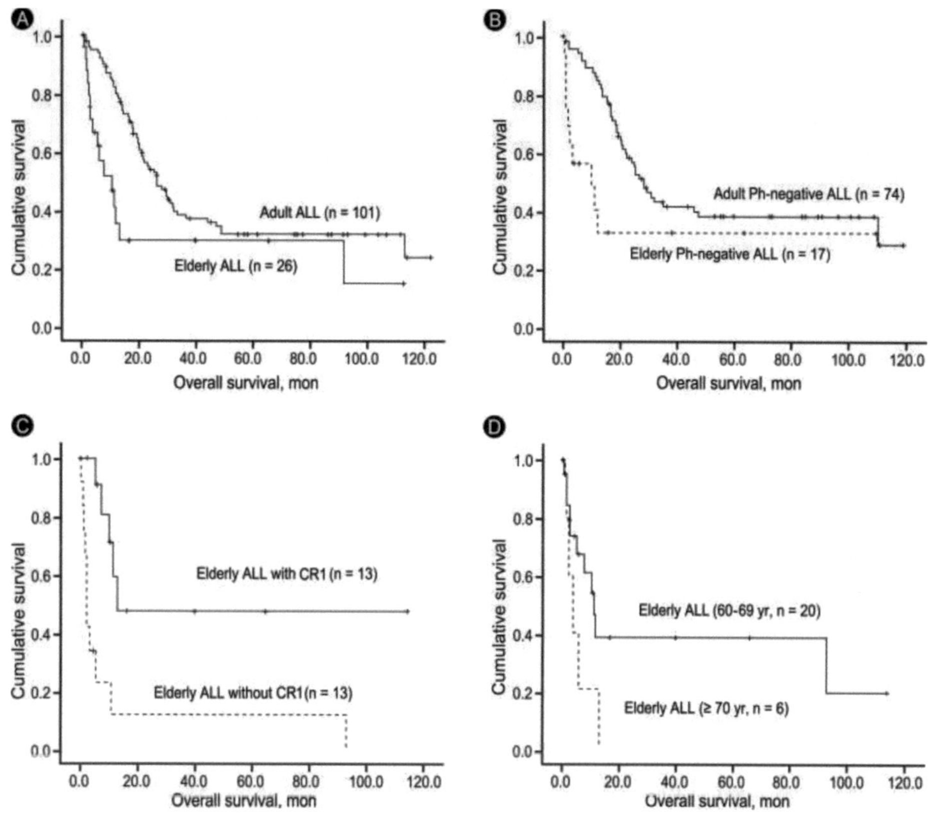

A. Overall survival (OS) of elderly and younger adult patients with acute lymphoblastic leukemia (ALL): OS of elderly patients with ALL (≥60 year) was shorter than that of younger adult patients with ALL (<60 year) (median OS 10.3 vs. 26.3 months, respectively, p = 0.003).

B. OS of the elderly and younger adult patients with Philadelphia chromosome (Ph)-negative ALL: OS of the elderly patients with Ph-negative ALL (≥60 year) was shorter than that of adult patients with Ph-negative ALL (<60 year) (median OS, 10.3 vs. 29.2 months, respectively, p = 0.01).

C. OS according to complete remission in elderly patients with ALL: OS of elderly patients with complete remission was longer than that of elderly patients without complete remission (median OS, 13.1 vs. 2.6 months, p = 0.001).

D. OS according to age (60–69 vs. ≥70 years) in elderly patients with ALL: OS of elderly patients aged 70 years or more was not significantly different from that of the other elderly patients (median OS, 11.2 vs. 3.7 months, p = 0.073) [40, 41].

8. Survival analysis for elderly patients with ALL

Among the elderly patients, the patients who achieved CR1 (CR after the first induction chemotherapy) showed significantly longer survival compared with those who did not achieve CR1 (median OS, 13.1 vs. 2.6 months; $p = 0.001$). Furthermore, CR1 was the only independent prognostic factor for OS in elderly patients with ALL ($p = 0.001$). Although the OS of elderly patients aged 60–69 tended to be longer than that of those aged 70 or over, the difference did not reach statistical significance (median OS, 11.2 vs. 3.7 months; $p = 0.073$).

In the survival analysis using the factors at the initial ALL diagnosis, the probable poor prognostic factors for CR were age ≥ 70 years (relative rate of remission [RR], 0.14; 95% CI, 0.013–1.45; $p = 0.098$) and leukocytosis (≥30,000/μL) (RR, 6.00; 95% CI, 0.93–38.63; $p = 0.059$). T-cell lineage and the presence of lymphadenopathy were significant factors in poor prognosis for OS in the univariate analysis (hazard ratio [HR], 3.11 and 3.14; 95% CI, 1.14–9.34, and 1.01–9.99; $p = 0.033$ and 0.041, respectively). T-cell lineage and Ph-positive status tended to increase the HR for leukemia free survival (LFS) (HR, 8.49 and 4.49; 95% CI, 0.53–135.82 and 0.8–25.21; $p = 0.069$ and 0.064, respectively).

Univariate analysis for complete remission, overall survival, and leukemia-free survival in elderly patients with ALL (≥60 year) (n = 26).

	Complete remission			Overall survival			Leukemia-free survival		
	RR	95% CI	*p* value	HR	95% CI	*p* value	HR	95% CI	*p* value
Age ≥ 70	0.14	0.013-1.45	0.098	2.60	0.88-7.67	0.073	4.48	0.41-49.46	0.18
T-cell lineage	0.22	0.019-2.53	0.23	3.11	1.14-9.34	0.033	8.49	0.53-135.82	0.069
Ph(+)	3.38	0.52-21.73	0.20	1.11	0.40-3.12	0.84	4.49	0.8-25.21	0.064
Lymph adenopathy	0.21	0.018-2.33	0.20	3.14	1.01-9.99	0.041	4.48	0.41-49.46	0.18
Male	0.50	0.09-2.73	0.42	1.80	0.57-5.64	0.31	1.13	0.20-6.26	0.89
Fever	1.67	0.13-21.20	0.69	0.84	0.19-3.72	0.82	0.033	0.00-253.78	0.22
WBC ≥ 30,000/μL	6.00	0.93-38.63	0.059	0.50	0.17-1.46	0.19	0.99	0.17-5.98	0.99

ALL, acute lymphoblastic leukemia; RR, relative rate of remission; CI, confidence interval; HR, hazard ratio; Ph, Philadelphia chromosome; WBC, white blood cell.

The low response to chemotherapy in the elderly patients with ALL could be related to several factors. The first factor may be chemotherapy intensity. Intensified combination induction chemotherapy can result in an improvement in the CR proportion, and high-dose postremission methotrexate (MTX) or cytarabine therapy is effective for treating adult ALL. However, most elderly patients with ALL in our study could not receive the postremission therapy after the induction therapy with a standard or reduced dose and also could not be treated with intensified postremission regimens such as cyclophosphamide or MTX, though they received postremission therapy. The second factor may be drug-resistance mechanisms such as the presence of multidrug-resistance gene 1 and multidrug-resistance-related protein.

Although intensified induction chemotherapy was not introduced, and postremission therapy was not performed appropriately in most elderly patients with ALL, the survival benefit was definite in the patients who achieved CR. Our study did not show a statistical difference in nondisease-related mortality rates between the elderly and younger adult groups. However, the actual risk of nondisease-related mortality might be significantly higher in the elderly patients considering that only a few patients could receive highly toxic therapy such as HSCT, and our results indicated that about half (43.8%) of nondisease-related mortality was related to HSCT in the younger adult patients with ALL [40–43].

8.1 New treatment options in older patients with ALL

ALL blasts express a number of antigens, such as CD33, CD22, CD19, and CD52, which could be targets for antibody therapy. The majority of older patients suffer from B-precursor ALL. In this subtype, approximately half of the patients show CD20 expression on their blast cells. In younger patients with $CD20^+$ ALL, the first promising data for the combination of chemotherapy and rituximab have been reported. Outcome of older patients could be hampered by a higher mortality due to infections in CR, which underlines the need for intensive supportive care for older patients throughout the entire treatment period.

A great majority of cases with ALL in elderly patient correspond to B-precursor lineage, one of the characteristics of this lineage is the expression of CD20 on its surface, which makes it susceptible to treatments focused on this marker, such as rituximab, this treatment approach has already shown to be highly effective in young patients, which could be transposed to the population over 65 years of age.

A promising new approach is the administration of a bispecific CD19 antibody, blinatumomab, which has the potential to engage cytotoxic T cells in patients for lysis of $CD19^+$ leukemia cells. In 19 patients with refractory disease, defined as hematologic remission with persistent MRD after intensive chemotherapy, the molecular remission rate was 84%. A number of older patients who were not able to receive an SCT remained in remission for more than 1 year. More recently, a CR rate of 68% was reported for relapsed ALL. All patients with CR also achieved a molecular CR. Treatment with the final dosing regimen was well tolerated, and a number of older patients experienced a benefit. The CD22 directed, calicheamicin-conjugated antibody inotuzumab induced 18% CRs and 39% marrow CRs in relapsed $CD22^+$ ALL. Toxicity appeared to be manageable, and the mortality of 4% within 4 weeks was moderate. Successful future use of antibody treatment will certainly depend on well-designed combination regimens with chemotherapy that aim to achieve long-term responses, particularly in older ALL patients.

In recent years, there have been advances and new therapeutic options in the management of ALL, one of the most promising is immunotherapy, specifically bispecific antibodies, the first of which useful information was disclosed was blinatumomab, this antibody that acts by binding to T lymphocytes, activating them and forcing them to destroy CD19 receptor expressing cells, such as blasts, already has multiple studies in various population groups that demonstrate their effectiveness against the disease, achieving significant response rates (84%) and negativization of the MRD. Another new specific antibody against the CD22 receptor, inotuzumab, has also been shown to be effective, at least in its initial studies, with a tolerable safety profile. The great advantage of these new treatments is that they do not confer the implicit risk in chemotherapy; however, there are no studies specifically in elderly patients.

Several other new drugs are of interest for optimizing treatment in older ALL patients. Although the number of older patients with T-ALL is low, the use of nelarabine is of interest after promising results and acceptable toxicity in relapsed T-ALL including older patients. Liposomal cytarabine for intrathecal application showed activity and tolerability in CNS relapse of ALL, although in combination with systemic neurotoxic regimens, severe toxicities may be observed. The use of liposomal cytarabine in prophylaxis of CNS relapse is of interest, particularly in older patients, since it allows reduction of the number of intrathecal injections and may induce fewer systemic toxicities compared to conventional intrathecal therapy.

Other drugs of current interest include nelarabine, indicated for use in cases of T-ALL. The prophylactic treatment to CNS has also had new protagonists in its field, liposomal cytarabine is one of these; this drug used for both prophylaxis and management of relapse to CNS has shown to be safe, although when combined with other neurotoxic agents, there is considerable toxicity. Despite this, safety is comparable to that presented by conventional cytarabine, with a higher rate of effectiveness.

Liposomal vincristine is another drug of interest, particularly in older patients. Results are still pending on the major question of whether liposomal encapsulation allows a higher dose intensity with lower risk of neurotoxicity. Bendamustine could be of interest, since it has shown limited toxicity and favorable results in older patients with B-cell lymphoma. New drugs with different mechanisms of action may, in the future, be used in combination with chemotherapy, such as proteasome inhibitors, histone-deacetylase inhibitors, hypomethylating agents, or targeted drugs such as Flt3 inhibitors or Jak2-inhibitors in defined subgroups of ALL. Currently, these compounds are either available in clinical trials or could be considered in individual patients with poor response to standard chemotherapy, including patients with molecular failure [12, 23, 43, 44].

Bendamustine and liposomal vincristine are new tools already known, the first one, a drug developed in the 1960s, has shown its effectiveness in various studies in the management of ALL and other lymphoproliferative disorders, with adequate safety in elderly patients. New mechanisms of action must be explored in order to give variety to the maneuvers against the disease. The study of new prognostic and risk markers that can be targeted by these drugs is crucial for their development. Currently, a large number of studies are underway in the world, both with new combinations of already known drugs and with novel molecules applicable to ALL [12, 23, 43, 44].

9. Conclusion

All older ALL patients need a comprehensive diagnostic classification, including, at least, immunophenotyping, molecular diagnostics, and setup of an assay for MRD evaluation. The identification of Ph+ ALL is crucial since, even in very old and frail patients, TKIs induce a high CR rate with reasonable durability. Furthermore, the biological characterization of older ALL patients needs to be improved. Biobanking for future scientific investigations within clinical trials should therefore be standard in older as it is in younger patients.

Altogether, in older as in younger patients, a pediatric-based induction strategy is recommendable in Ph− ALL. Dose reductions for anthracyclines are essential, and asparaginase during induction cannot be recommended outside of clinical trials. Dexamethasone appears to increase efficacy in younger patients, but prolonged use should be avoided. For fit older patients, consolidation chemotherapy may be intensified. Moderate-dose consolidation, including methotrexate, cytarabine, and reinduction therapy, appears to be feasible, and maintenance treatment is an essential treatment element.

In unfit older patients, a dose-reduced induction therapy is recommended with the aim of controlling and achieving a prolonged low-level disease. ALL-specific approaches should be considered, including vincristine, steroids, intrathecal therapy, and maintenance with mercaptopurine and methotrexate. Many physicians have more experience with older AML patients; however, there is no rationale for using AML regimens such as low-dose cytarabine or hydroxyurea in ALL.

When they are available, targeted drugs such as nelarabine, monoclonal antibodies, or other new drugs with potentially reduced or alternative toxicity should be added to treatment strategies in older patients, preferably in clinical trials. Since many of these compounds are used off-label, it may be useful to make the indication based on persistent MRD, which, in addition, offers a chance to evaluate effects immediately. Treatment options may change as soon as new drugs or strategies become available. With effective drugs for prolonged maintenance, it may be possible to further reduce intensity of induction therapy and avoid early mortality in unfit patients.

In Ph+ ALL, it is still not clear whether further reduced induction chemotherapy adds an effect to TKI therapy and which inhibitor is preferable. I favor a combination therapy. Moderate dose consolidation and maintenance should be offered. Patients should be considered as candidates for RIC SCT.

Whereas full-conditioning regimens before SCT are clearly not recommended, RIC SCT is an option in older patients. For indication, it will be crucial to define prognostic factors. Because persistence of MRD is one of the most important risk factors, MRD evaluation should take place in older patients to identify those who could benefit from experimental therapies or SCT. This also applies to Ph+ ALL regarding the option of changing the TKI.

Author details

Martha Alvarado Ibarra* and Jose Antonio De La Peña Celaya
Hematologists at Centro Médico Nacional "20 de Noviembre", ISSSTE Mexico City, Mexico

*Address all correspondence to: normoblasto@gmail.com

References

[1] Virgilio JF, Moscinski LC, Ballerter OF, et al. Acute lymphocytic leukemia ALL in elderly patients. Hematological Oncology. 1993;**11**:121-126

[2] Thomas DA, Giles FJ, Cortes J, et al. Antiangiogenic therapy in leukemia. Acta Haematologica. 2001;**106**:190-207

[3] Faderl S, Jeha S, Kantarjian HM. The biology and therapy of adult acute lymphoblastic leukemia. Cancer. 2003;**98**:1337-1354

[4] Miller MD, Towers A. A Manual of Guidelines for Scoring the Cumulative Illness Rating Scale for Geriatrics. Pittsburgh, PA: University of Pittsburgh; 1991

[5] Gökbuget N. Treatment of older patients with acute lymphoblastic leukemia. Hematology. American Society of Hematology. Education Program. 2016;**1**:573-579

[6] Gökbuget N. How I treat older patients with ALL. Blood. 2013;**122**:1366-1375

[7] Alvarado Ibarra M, Aguilar Andrade C, Báez Islas Pamela E, Cervantes Sánchez I, Chávez Aguilar Lénica A, Choque Condori Diana I, et al. Meeting report: Institute for social security and services for state workers (ISSSTE) on acute lymphoblastic leukaemia, México City, México, 3rd to 4th October 2016. International Journal of Medical Research & Health Sciences. 2017;**6**(6):21-69

[8] Moorman AV, Harrison CJ, Buck GA, et al. Karyotype is an independent prognostic factor in adult acute lymphoblastic leukemia (ALL): Analysis of cytogenetic data from patients treated on the Medical Research Council (MRC) UKALLXII/Eastern Cooperative Oncology Group (ECOG) 2993 trial. Blood. 2007;**109**:3189-3197

[9] Goldstone AH, Rowe J. How I treat acute lymphoblastic leukaemia. Blood. 2007;**110**:2268-2275

[10] Payne KJ, Dovat S. Ikaros and tumor suppression in acute lymphoblastic leukemia. Critical Reviews in Oncogenesis. 2011;**16**(1-2):3-12

[11] De Boer R, Koval G, Mulkey F, et al. Clinical impact of ABL1 kinase domain mutations and IKZF1 deletion in adults under age 60 with Philadelphia chromosome-positive (Ph1) acute lymphoblastic leukemia (ALL): Molecular analysis of CALGB (Alliance) 10001 and 9665. Leukemia & Lymphoma. 2016. [published online ahead of print]

[12] Jabbour E, O'Brien S, Ravandi F, Kantarjian H. Monoclonal antibodies in acute lymphoblastic leukemia. Blood. 2015;**125**(26):4010-4016

[13] Marks DI, Pérez WS, He W, et al. Unrelated donor transplants in adults with Philadelphia-negative acute lymphoblastic leukemia in first complete remission. Blood. 2008;**112**:426-434

[14] Ribera JM, Garcia O, Oriol A, PETHEMA Group, Spanish Society of Hematology, et al. Feasibility and results of subtype-oriented protocols in older adults and fit elderly patients with acute lymphoblastic leukemia: Results of three prospective parallel trials from the PETHEMA group. Leukemia Research. 2016;**41**:12-20

[15] Annino L, Goekbuget N, Delannoy A. Acute lymphoblastic leukemia in the elderly. The Hematology Journal. 2002;**3**(5):219-223

[16] Thomas DA, O'Brien S, Jorgensen JL, et al. Prognostic significance of CD20 expression in adults with de novo precursor B-lineage acute lymphoblastic leukemia. Blood. 2009;**113**:6330-6337

[17] Abdulwahab A, Sykes J, Kamel-Reid S, Chang H, Brandwein JM. Therapy-related acute lymphoblastic leukemia is more frequent than previously recognized and has a poor prognosis. Cancer. 2012;**118**(16):3962-3967

[18] Schwartz P, Hunault-Berger M, Chevallier PL, et al. French results with the EWALL chemotherapy backbone in older patients with Philadelphia chromosome-negative acute lymphoblastic leukemia. A GRAALL report. [Abstract]. Haematologica. 2013;**98**(S1):463. Abstract S1124

[19] Sabina C, Gina Z, Renato B. Diagnosis and subclassification of acute lymphoblastic leukemia. Mediterranean Journal of Hematology and Infectious Diseases. 2014;**6**(1):e2014073

[20] Brüggemann M, Schrauder A, Raff T, European Working Group for Adult Acute Lymphoblastic Leukemia (EWALL), International Berlin-Frankfurt-Münster Study Group (I-BFMSG), et al. Standardized MRD quantification in European ALL trials: Proceedings of the Second International Symposium on MRD assessment in Kiel, Germany, 18-20 September 2008. Leukemia. 2010;**24**(3):521-535

[21] Marks DI, Wang T, Perez WS, et al. Comparison of outcomes for non myeloablative and myeloablative conditioning for adults with ALL in first and second complete remission [abstract 872]. Blood. 2009;**114**:359

[22] Wetzler M, Sanford BL, Kurtzberg J, et al. Effective asparagine depletion with pegylated asparaginase results in improved outcomes in adult acute lymphoblastic leukemia: Cancer and Leukemia Group B Study 9511. Blood. 2007;**109**:4164-4167

[23] Thomas DA, O'Brien S, Kantarjian HM. Monoclonal antibody therapy with rituximab for acute lymphoblastic leukemia. Hematology/ Oncology Clinics of North America. 2009;**23**:949-971

[24] Thomas DA, Faderl S, Cortes J, et al. Treatment of Philadelphia chromosome positive acute lymphoblastic leukemia with hyper-CVAD and imatinib mesylate. Blood. 2004;**103**:4396-4407

[25] Burmeister T, Schwartz S, Bartram CR, Gökbuget N, Hoelzer D, Thiel E, GMALL Study Group. Patients' age and BCR-ABL frequency in adult B-precursor ALL: A retrospective analysis from the GMALL study group. Blood. 2008;**112**(3):918-919

[26] Mullighan CG, Williams RT, Downing JR, Sherr CJ. Failure of CDKN2A/B (INK4A/B-ARF)-mediated tumor suppression and resistance to targeted therapy in acute lymphoblastic leukemia induced by BCR-ABL. Genes & Development. 2008;**22**(11):1411-1415

[27] Ottmann OG, Druker BJ, Sawyers CL, et al. A phase 2 study of imatinib in patients with relapsed or refractory Philadelphia chromosome-positive acute lymphoid leukemia's. Blood. 2002;**100**(6):1965-1971

[28] Delannoy A, Delabesse E, Lhéritier V, et al. Imatinib and methylprednisolone alternated with chemotherapy improve the outcome of elderly patients with Philadelphia-positive acute lymphoblastic leukemia: Results of the GRAALL AFR09 study. Leukemia. 2006;**20**(9):1526-1532

[29] Ottmann OG, Wassmann B, Pfeifer H, GMALL Study Group, et al. Imatinib compared with chemotherapy as front-line treatment of elderly patients with Philadelphia chromosome-positive acute lymphoblastic leukemia (Ph1ALL). Cancer. 2007;**109**(10):2068-2076

[30] Vignetti M, Fazi P, Cimino G, et al. Imatinib plus steroids induces complete remissions and prolonged

survival in elderly Philadelphia chromosome-positive patients with acute lymphoblastic leukemia without additional chemotherapy: results of the Gruppo Italiano Malattie Ematologiche dell'Adulto (GIMEMA) LAL0201-B protocol. Blood. 2007;**109**(9):3676-3678

[31] Rea D, Legros L, Raffoux E, Intergroupe Francais des Leuceemies Myeloides Chronique, Group for Research in Adult Acute Lymphoblastic Leukemia, et al. High-dose imatinib mesylate combined with vincristine and dexamethasone (DIV regimen) as induction therapy in patients with resistant Philadelphia-positive acute lymphoblastic leukemia and lymphoid blast crisis of chronic myeloid leukemia. Leukemia. 2006;**20**(3):400-403

[32] Santos FP, Cortes J. Dasatinib for the treatment of Philadelphia chromosome-positive leukemias. Expert Opinion on Pharmacotherapy. 2012;**13**(16):2381-2395

[33] Benjamini O, Dumlao TL, Kantarjian H, et al. Phase II trial of hyper CVAD and dasatinib in patients with relapsed Philadelphia chromosome positive acute lymphoblastic leukemia or blast phase chronic myeloid leukemia. American Journal of Hematology. 2014;**89**(3):282-287

[34] Bergeron A, Rea D, Levy V, et al. Lung abnormalities after dasatinib treatment for chronic myeloid leukemia: A case series. American Journal of Respiratory and Critical Care Medicine. 2007;**176**(8):814-818

[35] Foá R, Vitale A, Vignetti M, GIMEMA Acute Leukemia Working Party, et al. Dasatinib as first-line treatment for adult patients with Philadelphia chromosome-positive acute lymphoblastic leukemia. Blood. 2011;**118**(25):6521-6528

[36] Ravandi F, O'Brien SM, Cortes JE, et al. Long-term follow-up of a phase 2 study of chemotherapy plus dasatinib for the initial treatment of patients with Philadelphia chromosome-positive acute lymphoblastic leukemia. Cancer. 2015;**121**(23):4158-4164

[37] Porkka K, Koskenvesa P, Lundan T, et al. Dasatinib crosses the blood-brain barrier and is an efficient therapy for central nervous system Philadelphia chromosome-positive leukemia. Blood. 2008;**112**(4):1005-1012

[38] Ravandi F, Jorgensen JL, Thomas DA, et al. Detection of MRD may predict the outcome of patients with Philadelphia chromosome-positive ALL treated with tyrosine kinase inhibitors plus chemotherapy. Blood. 2013;**122**(7):1214-1221

[39] Chalandon Y, Thomas X, Hayette S, Group for Research on Adult Acute Lymphoblastic Leukemia (GRAALL), et al. Randomized study of reduced-intensity chemotherapy combined with imatinib in adults with Ph-positive acute lymphoblastic leukemia. Blood. 2015;**125**(24):3711-3719

[40] Shah NP, Guilhot F, Cortes JE, et al. Long-term outcome with dasatinib after imatinib failure in chronic-phase chronic myeloid leukemia: Follow up of a phase 3 study. Blood. 2014;**123**(15):2317-2324

[41] Soverini S, Vitale A, Poerio A, et al. Philadelphia positive acute lymphoblastic leukemia patients already harbor BCR-ABL kinase domain mutations at low levels at the time of diagnosis. Haematologica. 2011;**96**(4):552-557

[42] Pfeifer H, Lange T, Wystub S, et al. Prevalence and dynamics of bcr-abl kinase domain mutations during imatinib treatment differ in patients with newly diagnosed and recurrent bcr-abl positive acute

lymphoblastic leukemia. Leukemia. 2012;**26**(7):1475-1481

[43] Jabbour E, Kantarjian H, Ravandi F, et al. Combination of hyper-CVAD with ponatinib as first-line therapy for patients with Philadelphia chromosome-positive acute lymphoblastic leukaemia: A single-centre, phase 2 study. The Lancet Oncology. 2015;**16**(15):1547-1555

[44] Le Jeune C, Thomas X. Potential for bispecific T-cell engagers: role of blinatumomab in acute lymphoblastic leukemia. Drug Design, Development and Therapy. 2016;**10**:757-765

Chapter 9

Neuromuscular Electrical Stimulation and Electromyographic Biofeedback as Adjunctive Modalities in the Treatment of Oropharyngeal Dysphagia in Stroke

Cláudia Tiemi Mituuti, Marcela Maria Alves da Silva and Giédre Berretin-Felix

Abstract

Dysphagia is a symptom related to swallowing disorders that impede or hamper safe, efficient, and comfortable oral ingestion. In addition to compromising the swallowing process, dysphagia may impair overall health, the nutritional status, and lung conditions, impacting quality of life as well. Different proposals for the rehabilitation of oropharyngeal dysphagia have been researched over the years. As a therapeutic strategy aimed at the rehabilitation of oropharyngeal dysphagias, the electromyographic (EMG) biofeedback provides improved strength in swallowing and its coordination, understood as the best muscle recruitment during the function, associated with the attention and performance of cortical functions, simultaneously. Neuromuscular electrical stimulation (NMES) is another therapeutic approach used in the rehabilitation of oropharyngeal dysphagia (NMES). NMES has been recommended as an adjunctive modality to improve the results of exercises based on dysphagia therapy. In view of the possibility of using technological resources in the diagnosis and treatment of oropharyngeal dysphagia, this chapter presents the theoretical and procedural framework aimed at the application of EMG biofeedback and NMES as supporting methods in the treatment of oropharyngeal dysphagia, in cases affected by stroke.

Keywords: dysphagia, stroke, rehabilitation, electromyography, neuromuscular electrical stimulation

1. Introduction

Dysphagia is a symptom related to swallowing disorders that impede or hamper safe, efficient, and comfortable oral ingestion [1], characterized by the abnormality in the transference of bolus from the mouth to the stomach [2]. In addition to compromising the swallowing process, dysphagia may impair overall health, the nutritional status, and lung conditions, impacting quality of life as well [3, 4].

IntechOpen

There are many neurological diseases that can affect the neural structures which control the complicated mechanisms of oropharyngeal swallowing. Most symptoms and complications from neurogenic dysphagia are due to sensory-motor change of the oral and pharyngeal phases of swallowing [5]. In adults and in the elderly population, dysphagia often derives from stroke [6].

Different proposals for the rehabilitation of oropharyngeal dysphagia have been researched over the years. Thus, literature review studies demonstrate the effectiveness of using protective and facilitating swallowing maneuvers, showing physiological changes in specific aspects of swallowing in normal subjects increasing or decreasing the pharyngeal contraction, the lingual pressure, the upper esophageal sphincter relaxation and contraction, according to the different techniques [7] and in the rehabilitation of oropharyngeal dysphagia reducing or eliminating aspiration and improving functional outcomes in specific populations [8, 9].

Orofacial myofunctional exercises are a therapeutic approach for the treatment of oropharyngeal dysphagia [10]. In poststroke individuals, tongue isometric exercises result in an increase in tongue force, with an associated improvement in swallowing pressure, airway protection, and tongue volume in acute or chronic phases [11].

In a late poststroke case, these tongue exercises were associated with improved bolus control and increased oral intake [12]. The use of surface electromyography (SEM) as a therapeutic biofeedback is a resource described in various areas of health, with studies showing clinical efficacy for a variety of neuromuscular disorders. The electromyographic biofeedback can be used to aid in muscle relaxation, coordination, and/or muscle response pattern training, as well as increased recruitment of motor units during muscular activity.

The McNeill Dysphagia Therapy Program (MDTP), which improves the timing of physiological events during swallowing, is another rehabilitation modality for patients presented with neurogenic dysphagia. Following MDTP, subjects presented with chronic dysphagia showed temporal coordination of swallowing components close to that of healthy individuals, thus suggesting a normalization of swallowing timing [13].

As a therapeutic strategy aimed at the rehabilitation of oropharyngeal dysphagias, the electromyographic biofeedback [14] provides improved strength in swallowing and its coordination, understood as the best muscle recruitment during the function, associated with the attention and performance of cortical functions, simultaneously [15, 16]. Its use has been described in cases of dysphagia due to stroke [17–20], as well as in cases of patients with sequelae from the treatment of head and neck cancer [19], with improvement in swallowing and consequent increase in the oral intake of patients treated with biofeedback associated with conventional therapy.

Neuromuscular electrical stimulation (NMES) is another therapeutic approach used in the rehabilitation of oropharyngeal dysphagia (NMES). NMES has been recommended as an adjunctive modality to improve the results of exercises based on dysphagia therapy. According to Wijting and Freed [21], NMES is the application of electrical current pulses to the skin to stimulate muscle contraction by peripheral motor nerves. The electric current causes a depolarization of the peripheral motor nerve, usually where the nerve enters the motor end plate, which, in turn, will elicit muscle contraction.

NMES has drawn the attention of speech therapists since the initial application for dysphagia by Freed et al. [22]. Some studies have shown improvement in swallowing physiology [22–24] and quality of life [25] after using NMES in individuals presenting with oropharyngeal dysphagia and also, specifically, in poststroke patients [26–28]. The increase in laryngeal excursion has been described as a physiological change in swallowing following NMES, related to the lowering of the hyoid bone during rest, in patients with neurogenic dysphagia [29, 30], and to the increase in the elevation of the larynx during swallowing [31].

In studies reporting higher level of oral intake [31, 32], decreased severity of dysphagia in patients with moderate dysphagia [33], increased sensitivity in poststroke individuals [34], and decreased laryngotracheal aspiration [31] were found as well. On the other hand, some studies found no difference in the clinical outcomes of patients undergoing rehabilitation with NMES, as compared to conventional therapy [35, 36].

In view of the possibility of using technological resources in the diagnosis and treatment of oropharyngeal dysphagia, this chapter presents the theoretical and procedural frameworks aimed at the application of EMG biofeedback and NMES as supporting methods in the treatment of oropharyngeal dysphagia, in cases affected by stroke.

2. Neuromuscular electrostimulation

Regarding the effect of NMEE on swallowing, there is not a uniform stimulation protocol in terms of duration, number of sessions, and parameters of the electric current. Some studies show positive results of NMES in the treatment of dysphagia, but others suggest negative effects on hyolaryngeal elevation or do not find differences with respect to conventional therapy. It is known that NMEE can directly modulate swallowing and interfere with the mechanisms of central control and execution. In addition, the closure of the vocal folds during swallowing and speech is modified by NMES, owing to weakness and paresis [37].

Additionally, the physiological responses obtained by NMEE can also be influenced by age and level of stimulation. A study [38] found interactions between age and stimulation amplitude on lingual and pharyngeal functions during swallowing. The anterior tongue pressure was reduced by motor stimulation in both age groups; however, the posterior lingual-palatal pressures were selectively reduced in adults. The base of tongue (BOT) pressures were increased by sensory stimulation in the elderly but decreased in young adults. Hypopharyngeal pressures were increased in both groups by motor stimulation. Therefore, age and NMEE level should be taken into account when planning the rehabilitation of swallowing disorders.

Specifically on the effectiveness of the application of NMES in poststroke dysphagia patients, several methods are proposed for NMES application, including level of stimulation, electrode placement, tasks requested during NMES, and frequency and duration of sessions. Aiming at understanding how the research has been conducted, **Table 1** presents the information on the studies that included poststroke individuals, in their samples.

Studies with patients suffering from stroke who used the sensory level of stimulation showed improvement in swallowing function and that the increase in the sensorial input to the cortex can reduce swallowing problems. The thyrohyoid muscle stimulation was used in most studies, using motor stimulation to increase the elevation of the larynx.

Stimulation of the thyrohyoid muscle was used in most studies, using motor stimulation to increase the elevation of the larynx. Most studies show positive effects of NMES in the performance of swallowing in patients presented with poststroke dysphagia, especially when the stimulus is applied at the sensory level or when the level of motor stimulation is applied to the infrahyoid muscles, during swallowing [45].

Research/authors	Beom et al. [39]	Kushner et al. [40]	Sun et al. [41]	Terré et al. [42]	Lee et al. [43]	Toyama et al. [44]
Stroke data	2.4 ± 2.1 months after stroke Cortex and subcortex	15.7 days after stroke Brain stem, brain hemisphere, and intracerebral hemorrhage	Brain stem and brain hemisphere	5 and 7 months after stroke	5.5 ± 2.1 day after stroke Cortical and subcortical Brain hemisphere	25.2 ± 25.9 weeks after stroke Hemorrhagic and ischemic
Age	66.1 ± 19.5 years	19–89 years	70.1 ± 8.9 years	32–71 years	63.4 ± 11.4 years	63.6 ± 21.4 years
Gender	3 males and 4 females	38 males and 27 females	24 males and 5 females	7 males and 2 females	22 males and 9 females	12 males
Stimulation level (device)	Tolerance (STIMPLUS DP200)	Tolerance (VitalStim)	Tolerance (VitalStim)	Tolerance (VitalStim)	120% of the mean of 3 tolerance threshold measures (VitalStim)	Motor (HPC device)
Electrode placement	Near the motor point of the digastric anterior belly muscle	Different for each patient	A pair, horizontally, above the hyoid bone and another, on the thyroid cartilage	A pair, horizontally, on the mylohyoid muscle and another on the thyrohyoid one	Infrahyoid region	Region of geniohyoid, mylohyoid, and digastric anterior belly muscles and thyrohyoid musculature
Tasks required	None	Exercises to increase strength, resistance, and amplitude of movement and mobility of the orofacial, lingual, and laryngeal musculature	Repeated effort swallowing	None	Tactile-thermal stimulation, tongue and closing-elevation larynx exercises, effort swallowing, and Mendelsohn, Masako, and Shaker maneuvers	3–10-minute NMES series, with 2-minute rest intervals, followed by conventional therapy with tongue exercises, tactile-thermal stimulation associated with dry effort swallowing, and Mendelsohn maneuver
Duration of sessions	30 minutes	60 minutes	60 minutes	45 minutes	30 minutes with NMES associated with conventional therapy	40 minutes
Number of sessions per week	5 sessions	5–6 sessions	5 sessions	5 sessions	5 sessions	5 sessions
Total of sessions	20 sessions	18 ± 3 sessions	12 sessions	20 sessions	15 sessions	40 sessions

DOI: http://dx.doi.org/10.5772/intechopen.84942

Research/authors	Beom et al. [39]	Kushner et al. [40]	Sun et al. [41]	Terré et al. [42]	Lee et al. [43]	Toyama et al. [44]
Exams carried out	Assessment by ASHA NOMS protocol and videofluoroscopy	FOIS	Clinical assessment, FOIS, and perceptive evaluation of swallowing ability by the visual analog scale	FOIS, patient's satisfaction scale, and videofluoroscopy, after and 3 months following therapy	FOIS and videofluoroscopy	FOIS, videofluoroscopy, and assessment of the anterior and upper displacements of the hyoid bone and larynx
Results	Improvement in the dysphagia and ASHA NOMS scales and in the videofluoroscopy	Improvement in the FOIS scale and better FOIS score, as compared to controls	Improvement in the FOIS scale and maintenance from 6 months to 2 years Improvement of the dysphagia degree and of the perceptive swallowing ability, following 6 months and stable after 2 years	Improvement in the FOIS and in the patient satisfaction scales Decrease of aspiration and of the delay in the triggering of the swallowing reflex	Improvement in the FOIS and swallowing function, in all periods	Improvement in the FOIS and dysphagia scales Greater anterior and upper displacement of the hyoid bone Greater upper laryngeal displacement in the experimental group

Table 1.
Information on the studies that included poststroke individuals, in their samples.

Thus, speech therapy sessions should be performed according to the selected therapy protocol, taking into account the characteristics of the patient's swallowing disorder and the goals to be achieved by the intervention.

Neuromuscular electrical stimulation is performed with a dual-channel electrotherapy system with an 80 Hz fixed current pulse and a 700 μs pulse duration (VitalStim, model 5900, Chattanooga Group), applied by a qualified professional.

Prior to placing the electrode in the skin, the anterior part of the neck should be cleaned with alcohol, so as to remove body oils that can interfere with the electrode contact. The placement of the electrodes used during therapy, for all participants, should meet their physiological needs of the patient. After placing the stimulation electrodes, the amplitude of the stimulation is increased by small increments.

The amplitude of the sensory and motor levels of NMES is determined based on the patient's description of the feeling, while the amplitude is increased from zero to the maximum tolerance. The minimum level of sensory stimulation is determined when the patient reports a tingling sensation, while the minimum motor level corresponds to sensation of tightness or pull [46].

The stimulation amplitude is set before therapeutic activities, individually determined at the motor or sensory levels, with functional tasks involving the swallowing of saliva or food of different volumes and consistencies, according to the possibility of safe feeding, identified by means of instrumental examination.

3. Surface electromyography and electromyographic biofeedback

Surface electromyography (SEMG) allows access to the physiological parameters of swallowing. Quantitative and qualitative analyses show that the normal swallowing in adults varies from individual to individual [47, 48] and is influenced by age. The pharyngeal phase is longer in children under 12 than in adults but with similar amplitude of muscle electrical signal [49], consistency, and bolus volume [50–52].

During electromyographic evaluation of swallowing, the activity of the suprahyoid muscles is 30–50% higher than that of the masseter muscles, and with advancing age, there is a decreased activity of the suprahyoid muscles and an increased masseter activity, with no statistically significant difference between men and women [47]. The literature has also shown a significant increase in the duration of muscle activity during swallowing, in patients over 70 years [53], and no difference between genders, both in the amplitude and duration of muscle activity, in the different age groups assessed [47, 53].

In addition to age, the use of dental prostheses influences the electromyographic activity. Authors [54] observed that, from the oral rehabilitation with implant-supported prostheses, the amplitude of the electromyographic signal for swallowing was the same found for dentate subjects, but the duration of muscle activity in this function is higher in users of prostheses. Authors [55] found a significant drop in activity for the masseter muscle following implant-supported oral rehabilitation in the elderly, resulting from the process of adaptation to the new conditions of stability generated by the fixation of total prostheses to the lower arch, in these subjects.

As an adjunctive method in the rehabilitation of oropharyngeal dysphagia, the electromyographic biofeedback can be used for the training of muscle relaxation, coordination, and/or muscle response patterns, as well as in the recruitment of a greater number of motor units during the activity of the stimulated muscle, in order to allow the patient to learn and monitor new muscle patterns using visual and/or auditory reinforcement [56, 57].

The application of electromyographic biofeedback in the treatment of dysphagia aims, primarily, at improving the swallowing strength and its coordination [16].

Studies show improvement in swallowing and, consequently, an increase in the oral intake of patients treated with biofeedback combined with conventional therapy [20, 24]. Research with this technique applied to swallowing disorders was initially carried out in a clinical case involving dysphagia of unknown etiology, which presented spasticity, rehabilitated with 20 sessions of EMG biofeedback and relaxation exercises to be done at home, with a significant improvement in the difficulty in swallowing, and maintenance of the results following 6 months of the end of the intervention [58].

The literature has shown improvement of swallowing in patients presented with poststroke neurogenic dysphagia, with an increased oral intake after the application of the biofeedback technique associated with conventional therapy, following seven training sessions [24] and after a 10-hour training carried out in a week [20], even in individuals previously rehabilitated with conventional exercises without success [20, 24]. A study [20] further reinforces that the functional improvement of swallowing was kept in six out of ten patients, up to 1 year after the intervention.

Another study examined the effectiveness of this technique in acute poststroke subjects using Mendelsohn's maneuver and EMG biofeedback for 2 weeks of rehabilitation and 2 weeks of non-rehabilitation, with groups which intercalated weeks of rehabilitation and non-rehabilitation and were assessed in each phase. In the rehabilitation week, the subjects were trained daily, twice a day, the first session being the learning of the maneuver and the remaining ones, training, during 30–40 swallowings. Significant changes were observed in hyolaryngeal duration and excursion (anterior and vertical), following the rehabilitation weeks [59].

Crary et al. [19] assessed the effectiveness of rehabilitation with EMG biofeedback in 25 patients presented with neurogenic dysphagia (poststroke) and in 20 subjects with mechanical dysphagia (posttreatment of head and neck cancer) in a 50-minute therapy, five times a week therapy, plus home training. All subjects improved their oral intake, with 92% improvement in neurogenic dysphagia and 80% in mechanics. Although the best result was seen in subjects presented with neurogenic dysphagia, they needed more sessions to complete the intervention, as compared to those with mechanical dysphagia.

Conventional therapy associated with electromyographic biofeedback should be performed during direct swallowing therapy, aiming at the learning of the new swallowing pattern. The strategies of the treatment with electromyographic biofeedback aim to achieve the neuromuscular adjustments required for the approximation of normal physiological patterns of the electromyographic recording, mainly of the suprahyoid muscles.

Additionally, the balance and coordination between different muscle groups, mainly those which elevate the jaw, orbicularis of the mouth, and suprahyoid muscles, can be approached, depending on the number of channels provided by the equipment. **Figure 1** illustrates the EMG biofeedback therapy.

The normal electromyographic pattern of swallowing and that performed by the patients should be presented to them, during the training, establishing a target track for functional training, in which the patients perform the enabling swallowing strategies, whose effectiveness must have been previously proven in the instrumental examination, aiming at approximating their neuromuscular recruitment to the normality physiological pattern, which involves, mainly, increasing the amplitude of the electromyographic signal of the suprahyoid muscles during function (greater muscle recruitment in the function). In addition, the functional training may aim at improving the coordination among other muscle groups involved in swallowing, increasing the recruitment of tongue muscle activity, in order to propel the bolus safely from the oral cavity through the pharynx, and increasing the amplitude of the muscle activity exerted during the effort of swallowing [16].

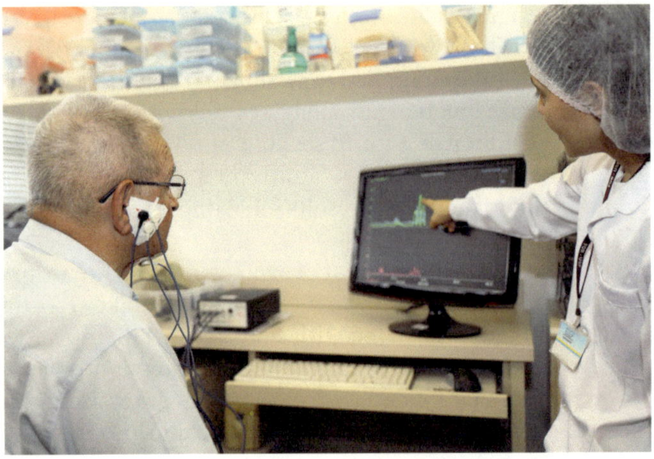

Figure 1.
Patient and therapist during the direct training of swallowing, using the EMG biofeedback (4-channel neuroeducation equipment), monitoring the masseters, bilaterally, and suprahyoid muscles.

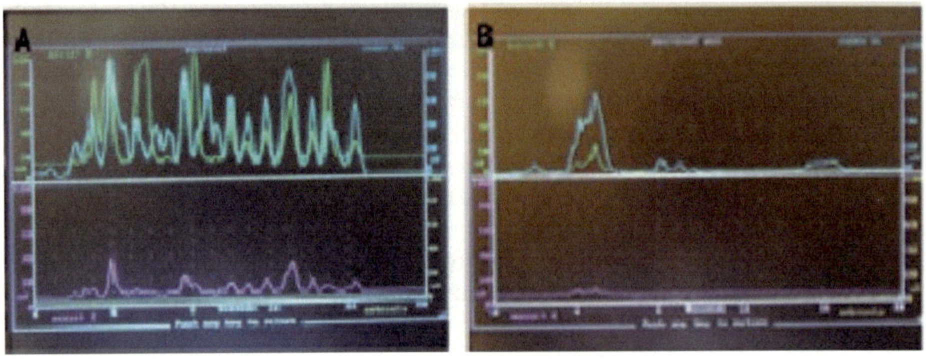

Figure 2.
(A) EMG signal prior to therapy. (B) EMG signal after therapy.

Figure 2A and **B** illustrate the neuromuscular behavior accomplished before and after a month of training, using biofeedback, whose sessions were held three times a week, in a patient presented with oropharyngeal neurogenic dysphagia with no success in the rehabilitation with conventional therapy.

The positive aspects of using the EMG biofeedback as an adjunctive method in cases of neurogenic dysphagia may pose this technique as a facilitator in terms of learning new neuromuscular patterns for swallowing, so as to provide the patient with a higher gain, as compared to the conventional therapy, as well as a probable longer effect of rehabilitation, since the EMG biofeedback involves the change of a previously learnt pattern, by means of the functional training therapy.

4. Conclusions

NMES has shown benefits in dysphagia therapy for individuals affected by stroke, mainly related to the classification of the degree of dysphagia and the level of oral intake. Some authors propose that the use of NMES associated with conventional therapy is more beneficial to the treatment of these individuals; however, there is a wide variety of electrode placement, level of the stimulus, and type and location of the stroke; thus, further studies are necessary to prove the efficacy of this treatment modality.

On the other hand, swallowing training using EMG biofeedback can assist speech therapists in their clinical practice, enabling the patient to learn and monitor new muscle patterns, using visual and auditory reinforcement, and, from the learning and training of new neuromuscular recruitment, present a swallowing pattern as functional as possible, with a positive impact on quality of life.

However, further controlled and randomized clinical studies are necessary for a understanding on the contribution of the EMG technique, for there are still many doubts on the application method, the number of therapeutic sessions, and the characteristics of patients who can benefit from the training with EMG biofeedback.

Conflict of interest

The authors declare no conflict of interest.

Author details

Cláudia Tiemi Mituuti[1]*, Marcela Maria Alves da Silva[2] and Giédre Berretin-Felix[3]

1 Federal University of Santa Catarina, Florianópolis, Brazil

2 Base Hospital of Bauru, Bauru, Brazil

3 Bauru School of Dentistry, University of São Paulo, Bauru, Brazil

*Address all correspondence to: claudia.mituuti@ufsc.br

References

[1] Alves NSG. O fundamental da avaliação fonoaudiológica do paciente disfágico. In: Costa M, Castro LP, editors. Tópicos Em Deglutição E Disfagia. Rio de Janeiro: Medsi; 2003. pp. 9-18

[2] Groher ME. Dysphagia: Diagnosis and Management. Boston: Butterworth-Heinemann; 1997

[3] Silva LM. Disfagia orofaríngea pós-acidente vascular encefálico no idoso. Revista Brasileira de Geriatria e Gerontologia. 2006;**9**(2):93-106

[4] Vale-Prodomo LP, Carrara-De-Angelis E, APB B. Avaliação clínica fonoaudilógica das disfagias. In: Geraldo Pereira J, Elisabete C-D-A, Ana Paula Brandão B, editors. Tratado da Deglutição e Disfagia: no Adulto e na Criança. Rio de Janeiro: Revinter; 2009. pp. 61-67

[5] Clavé ARLP. Videofluoroscopia y disfagia neurogénica. Revista Española de Enfermedades Digestivas. 2007;**99**(1):3-6

[6] Perlman AL. Disorderes swallowing. In: Tomblin JB, Morris HL, Spriesterbach DC, editors. Diagnosis in Speech—Language Pathology. San Diego, California: Singular Publishing Group; 1994. pp. 361-384

[7] Wheeler-Hegland K, Ashford J, Frymark J, McCabe D, Mullen R, Musson N, et al. Evidence-based systematic review: Oropharyngeal dysphagia behavioral treatments. Part II—Impact of dysphagia treatment on normal swallow function. Journal of Rehabilitation Research and Development. 2009;**46**(2):185-194

[8] Ashford J, McCabe D, Wheeler-Hegland K, Frymark T, Mullen R, Musson N, et al. Evidence-based systematic review: Oropharyngeal dysphagia behavioral treatments. Part III—Impact of dysphagia treatments on populations with neurological disorders. Journal of Rehabilitation Research and Development. 2009;**46**(2):195-204

[9] Silva RG. A eficácia da reabilitação em disfagia orofaríngea. Pró-Fono. 2007;**19**(1):123-130

[10] Burkhead LM, Sapienza CM, Rosenbek JC. Strength-training exercise in dysphagia rehabilitation: Principles, procedures, and directions for future research. Dysphagia. 2007;**22**(3):251-265

[11] Robbins J, Kays SA, Gangnon RE, Hind JA, Hewitt AL, Gentry LR, et al. The effects of lingual exercise in stroke patients with dysphagia. Archives of Physical Medicine and Rehabilitation. 2007;**88**(2):150-158

[12] Yeates EM, Molfenter SM, Steele CM. Improvements in tongue strength and pressure-generation precision following a tongue-pressure training protocol in older individuals with dysphagia: Three case reports. Clinical Interventions in Aging. 2008;**3**(4):735-747

[13] Lan Y, Ohkubo M, Berretin-Felix G, Sia I, Carnaby-Mann GD, Crary MA. Normalization of temporal aspects of swallowing physiology after the McNeill dysphagia therapy program. The Annals of Otology, Rhinology, and Laryngology. 2012;**121**(8):525-532

[14] Bryant M. Biofeedback in the treatment of a selected dysphagic patient. Dysphagia. 1991;**6**(3):140-144

[15] Nelson LA. The role of biofeedback in stroke rehabilitation: Past and future directions. Topics in Stroke Rehabilitation. 2007;**14**(4):59-66

[16] O'Kane L, Groher ME, Silva K, Osborn L. Normal muscular activity during swallowing as measured by surface electromyography. The Annals of Otology, Rhinology, and Laryngology. 2010;**119**(6):398-401

[17] Bogaardt HC, Grolman W, Fokkens WJ. The use of biofeedback in the treatment of chronic dysphagia in stroke patients. Folia Phoniatrica et Logopaedica. 2009;**61**(4):200-205

[18] Crary MA. A direct intervention program for chronic neurogenic dysphagia secondary to brainstem stroke. Dysphagia. 1995;**10**(1):6-18

[19] Crary MA, Carnaby-Mann GD, Groher ME, Helseth E. Functional benefits of dysphagia therapy using adjunctive sEMG biofeedback. Dysphagia. 2004;**19**:160-164

[20] Huckabee ML, Cannito MP. Outcomes of swallowing rehabilitation in chronic brainstem dysphagia: A retrospective evaluation. Dysphagia. 1999;**14**(2):93-109

[21] Wijting Y, Freed ML. VitalStim Therapy Training Manual. Hixson, TN: Chattanooga Group; 2010. p. 50

[22] Freed ML, Freed L, Chatburn RL, Christian M. Electrical stimulation for swallowing disorders caused by stroke. Respiratory Care. 2001;**46**(5):466-474

[23] Blumenfeld L, Hahn Y, LePage A, Leonard R, Belafsky P. Transcutaneous electrical stimulation versus traditional dysphagia therapy: A nonconcurrent cohort study. Otolaryngology-Head and Neck Surgery. 2006;**135**(5):754-757

[24] Bogaardt H, van Dam D, Wever NM, Bruggeman CE, Koops J, Fokkens WJ. Use of neuromuscular electrostimulation in the treatment of dysphagia in patients with multiple sclerosis. The Annals of Otology, Rhinology, and Laryngology. 2009;**118**(4):241-246

[25] Carnaby-Mann GD, Crary MA. Adjunctive neuromuscular electrical stimulation for treatment-refractory dysphagia. The Annals of Otology, Rhinology, and Laryngology. 2008;**117**(4):279-287

[26] Gallas S, Marie JP, Leroi AM, Verin E. Sensory transcutaneous electrical stimulation improves post-stroke dysphagic patients. Dysphagia. 2010;**25**(4):291-297

[27] Huang Z, Huang F, Yan HX, Min Y, Gao Y, Tan BD, et al. Dysphagia after stroke treated with acupuncture or electric stimulation: A randomized controlled trial. Zhongguo Zhen Jiu. 2010;**30**(12):969-973

[28] Xia W, Zheng C, Lei Q, Tang Z, Hua Q, Zhang Y, et al. Treatment of post-stroke dysphagia by vitalstim therapy coupled with conventional swallowing training. Journal of Huazhong University of Science and Technology. Medical Sciences. 2011;**31**(1):73-76

[29] Humbert IA, Polctto CJ, Saxon KG, Kearney PR, Crujido L, Wright-Harp W, et al. The effect of surface electrical stimulation on Hyo-laryngeal movement in normal individuals at rest and during swallowing. Journal of Applied Physiology. 2006;**101**(6):1657-1663

[30] Ludlow C, Humbert I, Saxon K, Poletto C, Sonies B, Crujido L. Effects of surface electrical stimulation both at rest and during swallowing in chronic pharyngeal dysphagia. Dysphagia. 2007;**22**(1):1-10

[31] Leelamanit V, Limsakul C, Geater A. Synchronized electrical stimulation in treating pharyngeal dysphagia. The Laryngoscope. 2002;**112**(12):2204-2210

[32] Permsirivanich W, Tipchatyotin S, Wongchai M, Leelamanit V,

Setthawatcharawanich S, Sathirapanya P, et al. Comparing the effects of rehabilitation swallowing therapy vs. neuromuscular electrical stimulation therapy among stroke patients with persistent pharyngeal dysphagia: A randomized controlled study. Journal of the Medical Association of Thailand. 2009;**92**(2):259-265

[33] Shaw GY, Sechtem PR, Searl J, Keller K, Rawi TA, Dowdy E. Transcutaneous neuromuscular electrical stimulation (VitalStim) curative therapy for severe dysphagia: Myth or reality? The Annals of Otology, Rhinology, and Laryngology. 2007;**116**(1):36-44

[34] Lim KB, Lee HJ, Lim SS, Choi YI. Neuromuscular electrical and thermal-tactile stimulation for dysphagia caused by stroke: A randomized controlled trial. Journal of Rehabilitation Medicine. 2009;**41**(3):174-178

[35] Kiger M, Brown CS, Watkins L. Dysphagia management: An analysis of patient outcomes using VitalStim-therapy compared to traditional swallow therapy. Dysphagia. 2006;**21**(4):243-253

[36] Bülow M, Speyer R, Baijens L, Woisard V, Ekberg O. Neuromuscular electrical stimulation (NMES) in stroke patients with oral and pharyngeal dysfunction. Dysphagia. 2008;**23**(3):302-309

[37] Miller S, Jungheim M, Kühn D, Ptok M. Electrical stimulation in treatment of pharyngolaryngeal dysfunctions. Folia Phoniatrica et Logopaedica. 2013;**65**(3):154-168

[38] Berretin-Felix G, Sia I, Barikroo A, Carnaby GD, Crary MA. Immediate effects of transcutaneous electrical stimulation on physiological swallowing effort in older versus young adults. Gerodontology. 2016;**33**(3):348-355

[39] Beom J, Kim SJ, Han TR. Electrical stimulation of the suprahyoid muscles in brain-injured patients with dysphagia: A pilot study. Annals of Rehabilitation Medicine. 2011;**35**(3):322-327

[40] Kushner DS, Peters K, Eroglu ST, Perless-Carroll M, Johnson-Greene D. Neuromuscular electrical stimulation efficacy in acute stroke feeding tube-dependent dysphagia during inpatient rehabilitation. American Journal of Physical Medicine & Rehabilitation. 2013;**92**(6):486-495

[41] Sun SF, Hsu CW, Lin HS, Sun HP, Chang PH, Hsieh WL, et al. Combined neuromuscular electrical stimulation (NMES) with fiberoptic endoscopic evaluation of swallowing (FEES) and traditional swallowing rehabilitation in the treatment of stroke-related dysphagia. Dysphagia. 2013;**28**(4):557-566

[42] Terré R, Martinell M, González B, Ejarque J, Mearin F. Treatment of oropharyngeal dysphagia with neuromuscular electrostimulation. Medicina Clínica. 2013;**140**(4):157-160

[43] Lee KW, Kim SB, Lee JH, Lee SJ, Ri JW, Park JG. The effect of early neuromuscular electrical stimulation therapy in acute/subacute ischemic stroke patients with dysphagia. Annals of Rehabilitation Medicine. 2014;**38**(2):153-159

[44] Toyama K, Matsumoto S, Kurasawa M, Setoguchi H, Noma T, Takenaka K, et al. Novel neuromuscular electrical stimulation system for treatment of dysphagia after brain injury. Neurologia Medico-Chirurgica. 2014;**54**(7):521-528

[45] Poorjavad M, TalebianMoghadam S, Nakhostin Ansari N, Daemi M. Surface electrical stimulation for treating swallowing disorders after stroke: A review of the stimulation intensity levels and the electrode placements. Stroke Research and Treatment. 2014;**2014**:918057

[46] Berretin-Felix G. Efeitos da estimulação elétrica neuromuscular na função de deglutição em jovens e idosos saudáveis. Bauru, SP: Livre-Docência, Faculdade de Odontologia de Bauru, USP; 2011

[47] Vaiman M, Eviatar E, Segal S. Surface electromyographic studies of swallowing in normal subjects: A review of 440 adults. Report 2. Quantitative data: Amplitude measures. Otolaryngology and Head and Neck Surgery. 2004;**131**(5):773-780

[48] Vaiman M, Eviatar E, Segal S. Surface electromyographic studies of swallowing in normal subjects: A review of 440 adults. Report 3. Qualitative data. Otolaryngology and Head and Neck Surgery. 2004;**131**(6):977-985

[49] Vaiman M, Segal S, Eviatar E. Surface electromyographic studies of swallowing in normal children, age 4-12 years. International Journal of Pediatric Otorhinolaryngology. 2004;**68**:65-73

[50] Perlman AL, Palmer PM, McCulloch TM, Vandaele DJ. Electromyographic activity from human laryngeal, pharyngeal, and submental muscles during swallowing. Journal of Applied Physiology. 1999;**86**:1663-1669

[51] Pernambuco Lde A, Silva HJ, Lima LM, Cunha RA, Santos Vda S, Cunha DA, et al. Electrical activity of masseter muscle in young adults during swallowing of liquid. Jornal da Sociedade Brasileira de Fonoaudiologia. 2011;**23**(3):214-219

[52] Ruark JL, McCullough GH, Peters RL, Moore CA. Bolus consistency and swallowing in children and adults. Dysphagia. 2002;**17**(1):24-33

[53] Vaiman M, Eviatar E, Segal S. Surface electromyographic studies of swallowing in normal subjects: A review of 440 adults. Report 1. Quantitative data: Timing measures. Otolaryngology and Head and Neck Surgery. 2004;**131**(4):548-555

[54] Haraldson T, Ingervall B. Muscle function during chewing and swallowing in patients with osseointegrated oral implant bridges. An electromyographic study. Acta Odontologica Scandinavica. 1979;**37**(4):207-216

[55] Berretin-Felix G, Nary Filho H, Padovani CR, Trindade AS Jr, Machado WM. Electromyographic evaluation of mastication and swallowing in elderly individuals with mandibular fixed implant-supported prostheses. Journal of Applied Oral Science. 2008;**16**(2):116-121

[56] Berretin-Felix G, Silva MMA, Mituuti CT. Terapia fonoaudiológica em deglutição (como eu trato). In: Marchesan I, Silva HJ, Berretin-Felix G, editors. Terapia Fonoaudiológica em Motricidade Orofacial. São José dos Campos: Pulso; 2012. pp. 147-162

[57] Rahal A, Silva MMA, Berretin-Felix G. Eletromiografia de superfície e biofeedback eletromiográfico. In: Pernambuco LA, Silva HJ, LBR S, Magalhães HV Jr, RVA C, editors. Atualidades em Motricidade Orofacial. Rio de Janeiro: Revinter; 2011. pp. 49-58

[58] Haynes SN. Electromyographic biofeedback treatment of a woman with chronic dysphagia. Biofeedback and Self-Regulation. 1976;**1**(1):121-126

[59] Mccullough GH, Kamarunas E, Mann GC, Schmidley JW, Robbins JA, Crary MA. Effects of mendelsohn maneuver on measures of swallowing duration post stroke. Topics in Stroke Rehabilitation. 2012;**19**(3):234-243

Chapter 10

Postural Imbalance in the Elderly: Main Aspects

Natália Moya Rodrigues Pereira
and Marcos Eduardo Scheicher

Abstract

The aging of the population is an unprecedented world phenomenon. Numerous physiological changes occur with aging, and one of the most common situations is postural imbalance and, consequently, the occurrence of falls. Balancing is the process of controlling the body's center of mass with respect to its base of support and depends on the integration of sensory systems (visual, vestibular, and somatosensory) with the central nervous system (CNS). Each system is prone to deterioration with advancing age and is influenced by age-related diseases and use of some types of medications and polypharmacy. As with any good clinical evaluation, a detailed history and a thorough physical examination are essential to evaluate postural balance. The evaluation of balance must be done with tests that are quick and with relatively little equipment and training. The improvement of postural balance can be done in many ways, and exercises are a type of this treatment and can be done with video games or a treadmill, for example.

Keywords: aging, postural balance, sensory systems

1. Aging of population

The aging of the population is an unprecedented world phenomenon. The projections of the World Health Organization indicate that by 2050, all ages will increase by 35%, people aged 65–84 will increase by 164%, older people aged 85–99 will increase by 301% and centenarians will grow by 746% [1].

Increasing longevity also contributes to an aging population. Globally, life expectancy at birth is projected to increase from 69 years in 2005–2010 to 76 years in 2045–2050 and to 82 years in 2095–2100 [1] (**Figures 1** and **2**).

Physiological changes are observed with aging, increasing the risks of developing chronic diseases and dependence care. Auditory, visual, and movement problems may be present in people 60 years or older. In addition, some conditions such as dementia, heart disease, stroke, respiratory disorders, diabetes, and musculoskeletal conditions (osteoarthritis and back pain) are more frequent in this age group [2].

One of the most common situations for the elderly is postural imbalance and, consequently, the occurrence of falls, representing a significant health problem in older adults. Each year, approximately 30% of community-dwelling older people

IntechOpen

fall at least once and 10–20% fall twice or more [3]. The incidence among institutionalized older people is even higher, with a mean percentage of residents who fall each year of over 40% [4].

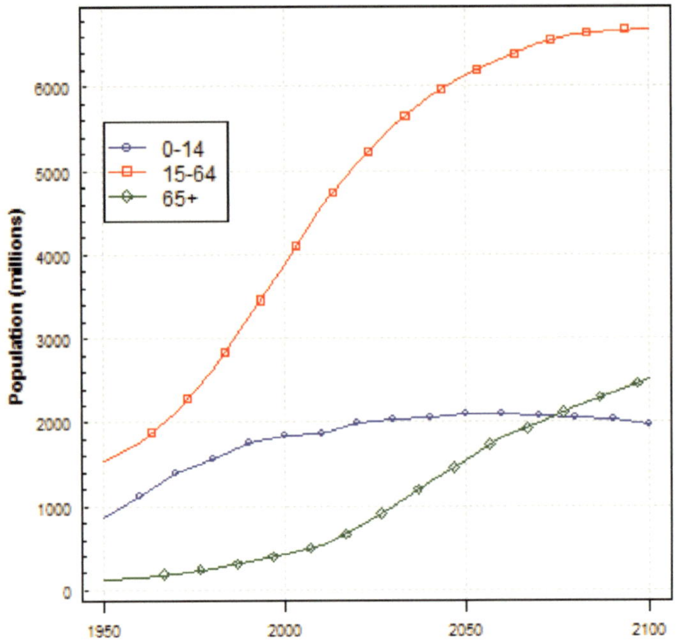

Figure 1.
Total population by broad age group. Courtesy: World Health Organization.

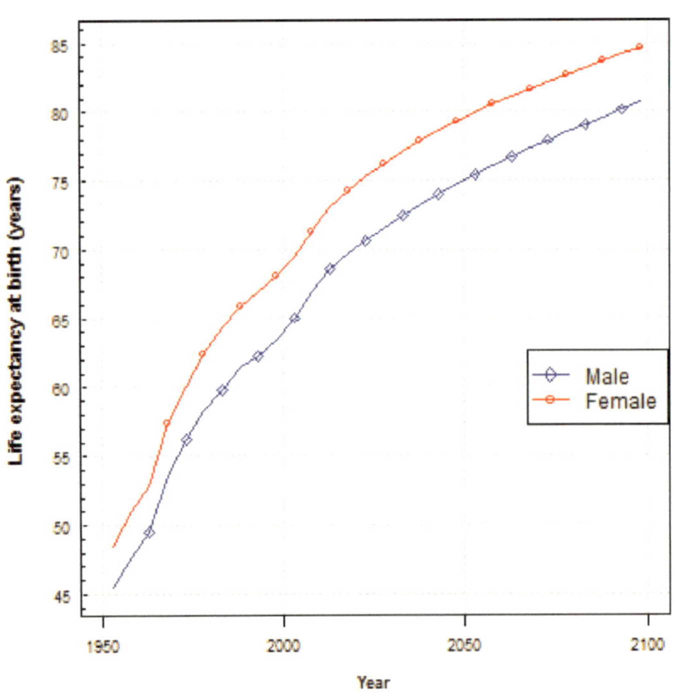

Figure 2.
Life expectancy at birth by sex. Courtesy: World Health Organization.

2. Postural balance

Balancing is the process of controlling the body's center of mass with respect to its base of support, whether in a static or dynamic situation. It depends on the integration of sensory systems with the CNS. Sensory information from somatosensory, visual, and vestibular systems must be integrated to interpret complex sensory environments. Each system interacts with each other to maintain balance in a closed loop, with an interrelation of cause and effect. When the sensory environment is changed, the CNS needs to re-weigh the contribution of each of the senses in postural balance. In an environment with good lighting and a firm surface, the contribution of somatosensory information is 70%, the visual information is 10%, and the vestibular information is 20% [5].

Each system is prone to deterioration with advancing age, and this is influenced by age-related diseases and use of some types of medications, in addition to polypharmacy [6]. Systems can partially compensate for each other's deterioration. Failing compensation strategies may eventually result in impaired balance, which may result in falls [7].

2.1 Vision and postural balance

The role of central and peripheral vision information in the control of movements and posture was examined in some studies [8, 9]. These authors suggested that peripheral vision is used for postural control and most particularly for stabilization of fore-aft sways, while the central vision is more often used for foot trajectory planning, targeting, obstacle avoidance, and stabilization of lateral sways.

Visual impairment is an important health problem and a major cause of injury in the elderly. Cataract, glaucoma, age-related macular degeneration, and diabetic retinopathy are the most common diseases related to the elderly and can interfere with the postural balance.

2.1.1 Cataract

Cataract, affecting mainly visual acuity and contrast sensitivity, contributes to about 50% of visual impairments in the elderly [10, 11]. The consequences include decreased ability to perform activities of daily living (such as reading, watching television, driving, and interacting socially), depression, increased number of falls, and increased mortality [10, 12]. The impact on patients is comparable with that of major systemic conditions including stroke, diabetes, and arthritis. In a study in patients with cataract, Pasma et al. found a higher proprioceptive weight compared with healthy elderly participants, which means that the elderly with cataract rely more on their proprioceptive information [7].

2.1.2 Glaucoma

Glaucoma is a progressive optic neuropathy characterized by degeneration of retinal ganglion cells and their axons with consequent vision loss and blindness. This condition leads to a characteristic reduction in the visual field (VF), with good central visual acuity. Previous studies have reported a higher risk of falling in patients with glaucoma compared to normal subjects [13–15]. In the study by Black et al., a cohort of glaucoma subjects was examined to assess body displacement of the trunk and the results showed that the worse the visual field defect, the greater the body sway [16].

2.1.3 Age-related macular degeneration

Age-related macular degeneration (AMD) is a disease that affects the macula (central vision), altering the accuracy of vision necessary for "direct" and fine activities, and may interfere with activities of daily living [17].

Wood et al. studied postural balance in older adults with AMD and showed that diminution of contrast sensitivity and visual field loss lead to postural instability and mobility difficulties in these patients [18]. Chatard et al., studying 10 elderly unilateral AMD subjects, 10 elderly bilateral AMD subjects, and 10 healthy age-matched control subjects, showed that bilateral AMD subjects had a surface area and an antero-posterior displacement of the CoP higher than healthy elderly. Unilateral AMD subjects had more antero-posterior displacement of the CoP than healthy elderly [19]. The authors conclude that because of aging, AMD subjects could have poor postural adaptive mechanisms which increase instability and risk of falls.

2.1.4 Diabetic retinopathy

Diabetic retinopathy (DR) is a common and potentially blinding microvascular complication of diabetes [20]. In a study, Gupta et al. found that diabetes per se was not a risk factor for falls. However, the authors found an association between diabetic patients with DR and risk of falling [20], suggesting a relation between DR and postural balance.

The greater tendency to fall in patients with mild-to-moderate DR can be explained by a reduction in the components of the visual function system, such as contrast, sensitivity, stereo acuity, and color perception [21, 22].

Figure 3 summarizes the normal vision and main eye disorders that can interfere with the postural balance described above.

Thus, it is important to evaluate visual function when we propose to work with postural balance in the elderly.

2.2 Vestibular system and postural balance

Through its sensory functions, the vestibular system detects the position and movement of the head in space relative to gravity, and helps to stabilize vision and balance [23].

The vestibular system has structures similar to miniaturized accelerometers, which report continuous information to the cerebral cortex, cerebellum, and somatic sensory cortices on the movements and position of the head and body. The vestibular nuclei make connections with structures of the brainstem and cerebellum and also innervate the motor neurons that control extraocular, cervical, and postural muscles [23] (**Figure 4**).

Impaired function of the vestibular system causes vertigo, loss of balance, and loss of gaze fixation during movement, often accompanied by dizziness and nausea [24].

Vestibular dysfunction is typically characterized by vertigo (i.e., an illusory sense of motion) and imbalance owing to disturbances in gaze and postural stability [25], which can culminate in falls [26].

So, the evaluation of the vestibular system is indispensable when the patients have a impaired balance control.

2.3 Somatosensory system and postural balance

People rely primarily on the proprioceptive and cutaneous input to maintain normal quiet stance and to safely accomplish the majority of activities of daily living [27].

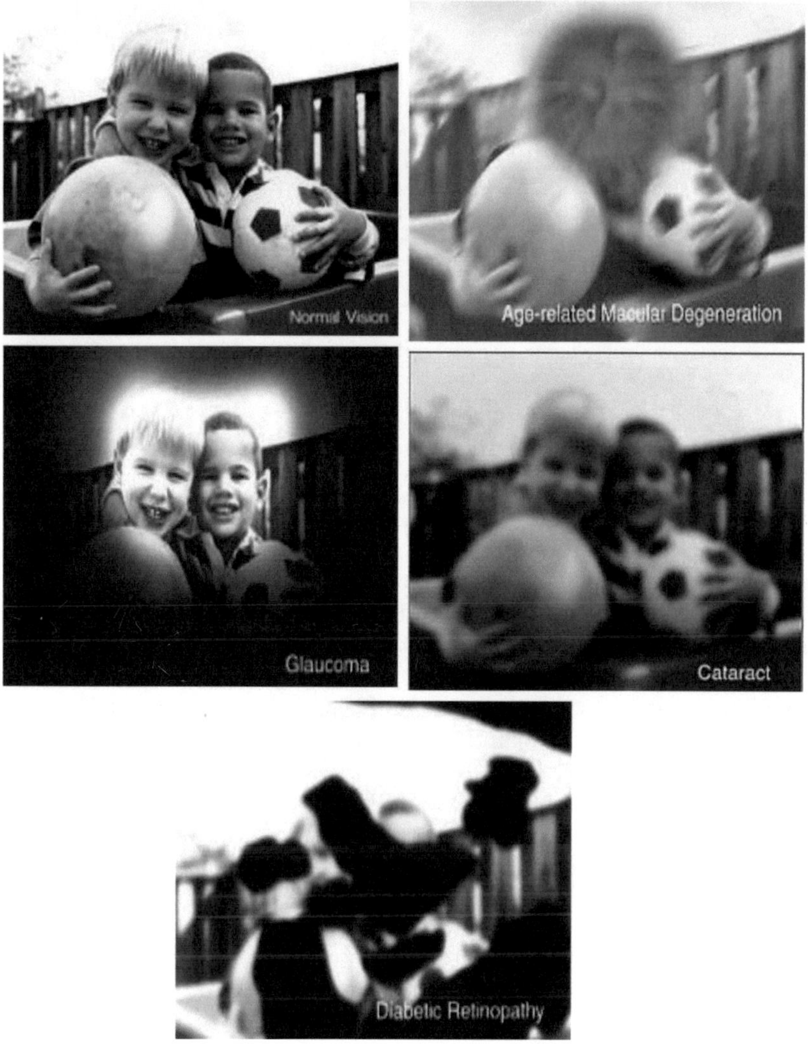

Figure 3.
The main vision impairments that interfere with balance. Courtesy: National Eye Institute, National Institutes of Health (NEI/NIH).

The proprioceptive information depends on muscle spindles, the Golgi tendon organ (GTO), and articular receptors. The first provide the nervous system with information about the muscle's length and velocity of contraction, thus contributing to the individual's ability to discern joint movement and position sense [28]. Besides, the muscle spindles provide afferent feedback that translates stimuli to appropriate reflexive and voluntary movements. The GTO relays information about tensile forces, and is sensitive to very slight changes [28], and when it is activated, the afferent neuron synapses in the spinal cord interneurons, which inhibit the muscle alpha motoneuron, resulting in decreased tension in muscle and tendon. Articular or joint proprioceptors respond to mechanical deformation of the joint capsule and ligaments.

On a slippery or dry floor surface, people show different gait parameters, including step length, required coefficient of friction, and heel contact velocity, evidencing the importance of the sensorimotor system in balance control [29].

Sensorimotor impairments occur with aging and are believed to contribute to the increased likelihood of imbalance and falling [30]. Damage to joint and muscular

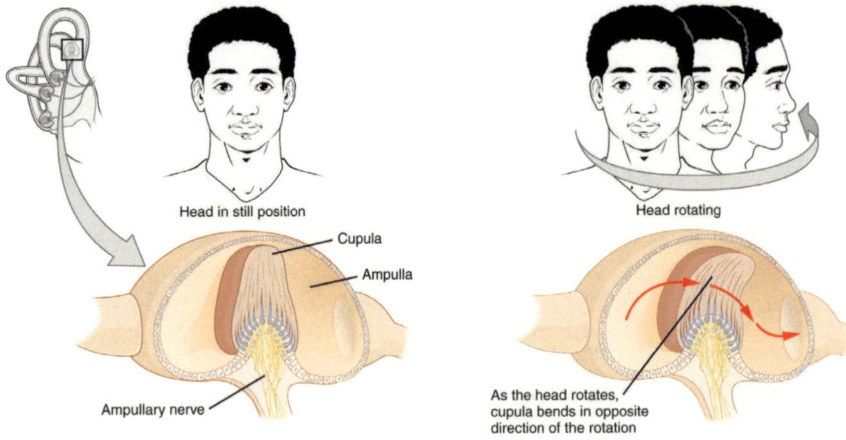

Figure 4.
Postural balance and the vestibular system responses. From Wikimedia Commons, https://commons.wikimedia.org/wiki/File:1410_Equilibrium_and_Semicircular_Canals.jpg.

proprioception, strength (capacity of muscle strength), and reaction time may contribute to the increase in the probability of fall [30].

Some diseases can affect muscles and joints. Studies have shown that, in patients with knee osteoarthritis (AO), postural balance is impaired due to reduced quadriceps function and decreased proprioception [31, 32]. Among elderly individuals, the prevalence of knee OA is approximately 12.2%, with a higher prevalence in women (14.9%) than in men (8.7%) [33].

Patients with neuromuscular diseases (NMDs), usually characterized by muscle weakness, appear to fall regularly. Aging causes a loss of muscle mass with a preferential decline in type II fibers [34], besides decrements in force production, power, specific tension, and fatigability [35], increasing the risk of falls.

Key points

- Elderly population is increasing.
- Postural imbalance and falling are serious problems faced by the older population.
- Postural control is based on the interpretation by central nervous system of convergent sensory information from somatosensory, vestibular, and visual systems.
- Impairments in these systems lead directly to functional loss, such as the inability to walk safely, to climb stairs, and dress independently, increasing the risk of falls.

3. Approach to the patient with a balance problem

3.1 Physical examination

As with any good clinical evaluation, a detailed history and a thorough physical examination are essential. As the postural balance depends on several systems, it is essential to evaluate the visual system, the vestibular and auditory system, and the sensorimotor system.

3.2 Functional performance tests

A comprehensive assessment of balance is important for both diagnostic and therapeutic reasons in clinical practice.

The tests can be divided between single-task measures and multiple-task measures [36]. These tests often can be done very quickly and with relatively little equipment and training.

3.2.1 Single-task measures

3.2.1.1 Single-leg stance test

The single leg-stance test (SLS) is simple, has high reliability and low cost, and is widely used for diagnosis and follow-up of patients in research and clinical settings. In this test, the participant remains supported on one leg, with arms resting on the hips, and the time (in seconds) that the patient remains in the position without unbalance is verified [37]. Decreased eyes-open SLS time is associated with an increased risk for falls [38].

3.2.1.2 Functional reach test

The *functional reach test* (FRT) is an easy and inexpensive test in which the patient flexes the trunk, extending the arms horizontally and keeping the feet in contact with the ground. The score is obtained by measuring the distance between the initial and the final positions of the fingertip [39]. Displacements less than 15 cm indicate postural balance problems and increased risk of falls [40].

3.2.1.3 Gait speed test

The *gait speed test* gives an easy, inexpensive, reliable measure of functional capacity [41], with high interrater and test-retest reliability [42]; does not require laboratory equipment; is not limited to a specific health care discipline [43]; and may be done quickly in clinical settings. The test may vary according to the pace (usual or maximal speed), whether static or moving start, and the distance walked (ranging from 4 to 500 m) [44].

3.2.2 Multiple-task measures

3.2.2.1 Berg Balance Scale

The *Berg Balance Scale* (BBS) consists of a battery of 14 tasks common to the activities of daily living, which quantitatively evaluate the risk of falls, through observations undertaken by the examiner [45]. The score on the test ranges from 0 to 56 and the performance on each task is measured on a five-point scale ranging from 0 to 4 (0 = unable to perform, 4 = independent). Scores of 48 or less indicate inability to walk independently and safely in activities of daily living and, consequently, increased risk of falls [46].

3.2.2.2 Short physical performance battery

The *short physical performance battery* (SPPB) is designed to measure functional status and physical performance, assessing walking speed, standing balance, and sit-to-stand performance [47]. The scores range from 0 (worst performance) to 12 (best performance). In a study, Veronese et al. demonstrated that SPPB scores ≤6 are associated with a higher fall rate in old people [48].

3.2.2.3 Timed up and go

The *Timed up and go* (TUG) test was developed in 1991 [49]. The test consists of finding the time the patient takes to get up from a chair (height about 46 cm), walk the distance of 3 m at a comfortable and safe step, turn around and go back to the chair, and sit down again. The subject wears his regular footwear and uses his customary walking aid (cane or walker) if necessary [49]. A faster time indicates a better functional performance [50].

Key points

- A good clinical evaluation, a detailed history, and a thorough physical examination are essential to evaluate postural balance.
- The tests can be divided between single-task and multiple-task measures.
- Assessment of balance is important for both diagnostic and therapeutic reasons in clinical practice.

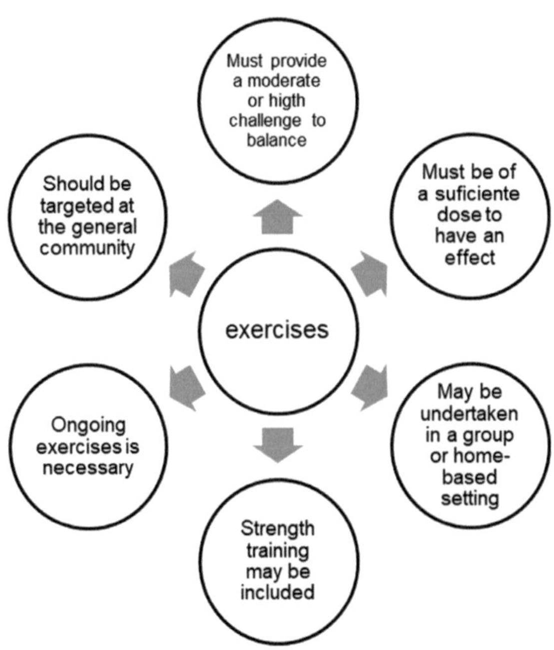

Figure 5.
Recommendations to guide the use of exercise for falls prevention.

4. Improvement of the postural balance

Falls are a public health problem. The risk of falling increases with age for many reasons, for example overall weakness and frailty, balance problems, cognitive problems, vision problems, some medications and polypharmacy, acute illness, and other environmental hazards. Because of this, multifactorial interventions should include an initial assessment of modifiable risk factors for falls and subsequent customized interventions for each patient based on issues identified in the initial assessment.

One type of treatment to improve balance is physical exercise. **Figure 5** presents a summary of best practice recommendations to use for improving postural balance and, consequently, fall prevention.

4.1 Types of exercises

Any physical exercise that overloads the balance systems without putting the patient at risk is recommended. It is possible, for example, to make a training circuit, with different stimuli for the elderly [51]. In the circuit, exercises such as one-legged support (both sides), gait on unstable surface, tandem gait, among others can be done, always increasing the level of difficulty.

Another possibility is to join two modalities of exercises: video games and muscle strengthening, for example. In a study, Prata and Scheicher found improvement in fear of falling and in mobility after 12 weeks of video game and muscle strength training in older women with a history of falls [52].

4.1.1 Video games

Postural balance training involving new technologies can promote more challenging situations for the elderly, increasing patient motivation and adherence to the program [53]. The use of video games provides immediate visual feedback, allowing users to make changes in motion according to the situations of the games and thus to develop strategies to restore and/or maintain postural balance, and may therefore be effective for the prevention of falls [54].

Carvalho et al. showed an increase in gait speed and a decrease in the TUG time in elderly female fallers after 12 weeks of training (two sessions per week) with commercialized games of Wii Fit by Nintendo® in sync with the Wii Balance Board® [55]. Three different games were used for postural balance training: *Penguin Slide*, where the participants had to catch fish while balanced on a piece of ice by shifting their weight from side to side; *Table Tilt*, where participants move their bodies in various directions to put balls into holes; and *Tightrope*, where participants walk on a tightrope with several vertical jumps to avoid obstacles.

4.1.2 Treadmill exercise

In the last decade, the use of the treadmill in the rehabilitation of gait in Parkinson's disease patients, stroke patients, and cerebral palsy (CP) patients has been studied. Some studies explain the reasons for improving postural balance patterns with treadmill training. One of them explains that treadmill training has the capacity to promote motor re-learning and, consequently, improve locomotor capacity during walking [56]. It has also been suggested that training, through repetitive movements generated by the treadmill, activates locomotor patterns of functional movements, sensory inputs, and circuits of the central nervous system [57]. In addition, it has been hypothesized that repetitive movements associated with cutaneous and proprioceptive impulses may induce activation of central movement patterns and, in the long term, potentiate the motor cortex, facilitating motor learning [58].

Toole et al. and Frenkel-Toledo et al. showed an improvement in the gait and balance in Parkinson's patients that participated in a six-week treadmill walking program [59, 60]. Herman et al. showed an enhancement in the gait rhythmicity and several improvements in motor signs, the latter remaining significantly better 4 weeks after the training was stopped [61].

Training on a treadmill to fight the stroke-related disabilities resulted in valuable results: fatigue resistance [62], endurance performance improvement [63], and the development of motor function [64]. A study in chronic non-ambulatory hemiparetic subjects revealed that partial body weight–supported treadmill training was superior to conventional physiotherapy with regard to restoration of gait and improvement of ground walking velocity [65]. In this study, during one 30-min session of treadmill training, patients could practice up to 1000 gait cycles as compared with a median of less than 50 gait cycles during one regular physiotherapy session.

Bjornson et al. studied the effect of short-burst interval locomotor treadmill training on walking capacity and performance in cerebral palsy and concluded that this training may improve short-term walking capacity and performance [66]. In another study, Mattern-Baxter et al. concluded that home-based treadmill training accelerates the attainment of walking skills and decreases the amount of support used for walking in young children with CP [67].

In healthy elderly with falls history, there are few studies that evaluated the responses of the postural balance with the treadmill training. Dorfman et al. found that after 6 weeks of treadmill plus dual-task training program, elderly fallers demonstrated improved scores on tests of mobility, functional performance tasks, and cognition [68]. In another study, van Ooijen et al., using a treadmill training with visual context, found improvement in walking ability and reduced risk of falls and fear of falling in older adults with a recent fall-related hip fracture [69].

Key points

- Any physical exercise that overloads the balance systems without putting the patient at risk is recommended.
- Postural balance training involving new technologies can promote more challenging situations for the elderly, increasing patient motivation and adherence to the program.
- Treadmill training is another form of exercise to challenge the postural control system.

5. Conclusion

It is necessary to consider the various facets of the postural balance system when a patient presents a problem related to this. Evaluating these facets is important in prescribing the correct treatment for each situation. There are many types of training that can improve postural balance. Physical exercises, when performed with a moderate or high challenge to the balance system, are a type of treatment that can help reduce the risk of falls in the elderly.

Conflict of interest

The authors declare no conflicts of interest.

Author details

Natália Moya Rodrigues Pereira[1] and Marcos Eduardo Scheicher[2]*

1 Biosciences Institute, UNESP, Rio Claro, São Paulo, Brazil

2 Physiotherapy and Occupational Therapy Department, UNESP, Marília, São Paulo, Brazil

*Address all correspondence to: marcos.scheicher@unesp.br

References

[1] United Nations. World population prospects: The 2012 revision. Highlights and advance tables. Population and Development Review. 2013;**36**:775-801. Available from: http://esa.un.org/unpd/wpp/Documentation/publications.htm

[2] World Health Organization. Integrated Care for Older People [Internet]. Geneva; 2017. 46 p. Available from: http://apps.who.int/iris/bitstream/10665/258981/1/9789241550109-eng.pdf?ua=1

[3] Graafmans WC, Ooms ME, Hofstee HMA, Bezemer PD, Bouter LM, Lips P. Falls in the elderly: A prospective study of risk factors and risk profiles. American Journal of Epidemiology. 1996;**143**(11):1129-1136. Available from: https://academic.oup.com/aje/article-lookup/doi/10.1093/oxfordjournals.aje.a008690

[4] Rubenstein LZ, Josephson KR. The epidemiology of falls and sincope. Clinics in Geriatric Medicine. 2002;**18**: 141-158

[5] Peterka RJ. Sensorimotor integration in human postural control. Journal of Neurophysiology. 2002;**88**:1097-1118

[6] Maki B, McIlroy W. Postural control in the older adult. Clinics in Geriatric Medicine. 1996;**12**(4):635-658

[7] Pasma JH, Engelhart D, Maier AB, Schouten AC, van der Kooij H, Meskers CGM. Changes in sensory reweighting of proprioceptive information during standing balance with age and disease. Journal of Neurophysiology. 2015; **114**(6):3220-3233. Available from: http://jn.physiology.org/lookup/doi/10.1152/jn.00414.2015

[8] Berencsi A, Ishihara M, Imanaka K. The functional role of central and peripheral vision in the control of posture. Human Movement Science. 2005;**24**(5–6):689-709

[9] Marigold DS, Patla AE. Visual information from the lower visual field is important for walking across multi-surface terrain. Experimental Brain Research. 2008;**188**(1):23-31

[10] Desapriya E, Subzwari S, Scime-Beltrano G, Samayawardhena LA, Pike I. Vision improvement and reduction in falls after expedited cataract surgery. Systematic review and metaanalysis. Journal of Cataract & Refractive Surgery. 2010;**36**(1):13-19. DOI: 10.1016/j.jcrs.2009.07.032

[11] Chew M, Chiang PPC, Zheng Y, Lavanya R, Wu R, Saw SM, et al. The impact of cataract, cataract types, and cataract grades on vision-specific functioning using rasch analysis. American Journal of Ophthalmology. 2012;**154**(1):29-38

[12] Polack S, Kuper H, Wadud Z, Fletcher A, Foster A. Quality of life and visual impairment from cataract in Satkhira district, Bangladesh. British Journal of Ophthalmology. 2008;**92**(8): 1026-1030

[13] Wood JM, Lacherez P, Black AA, Cole MH, Boon MY, Kerr GK. Risk of falls, injurious falls, and other injuries resulting from visual impairment among older adults with age-related macular degeneration. Investigative Ophthalmology & Visual Science. 2018; **52**(8):5088-5092

[14] Black AA, Wood JM, Lovie-Kitchin JE. Inferior field loss increases rate of falls in older adults with glaucoma. Optometry and Vision Science. 2011; **88**(11):1275-1282

[15] Coleman AL, Stone K, Ewing SK, Nevitt M, Cummings S, Cauley JA, et al. Higher risk of multiple falls among

elderly women who lose visual acuity. Ophthalmology. 2004;**111**(5): 857-862

[16] Black AA, Wood JM, Lovie-Kitchin JE, Newman BM. Visual impairment and postural sway among older adults with glaucoma. Optometry and Vision Science. 2008;**85**(6):489-497

[17] National Eye Institute. Age-Related Macular Degeneration (AMD) [Internet]. [cited 2018 Jun 26]. Available from: https://nei.nih.gov/health/maculardegen

[18] Wood JM, Lacherez PF, Black AA, Cole MH, Boon MY, Kerr GK. Postural stability and gait among older adults with age-related maculopathy. Investigative Ophthalmology and Visual Science. 2009;**50**(1):482-487

[19] Chatard H, Tepenier L, Jankowski O, Aussems A, Allieta A, Beydoun T, et al. Effects of age-related macular degeneration on postural sway. Frontiers in Human Neuroscience. 2017; **11**(March):1-9. Available from: http://journal.frontiersin.org/article/10.3389/fnhum.2017.00158/full

[20] Gupta P, Aravindhan A, Gan ATL, Man REK, Fenwick EK, Mitchell P, et al. Association between the severity of diabetic retinopathy and falls in an Asian population with diabetes the Singapore epidemiology of eye diseases study. JAMA Ophthalmology. 2017; **135**(12):1410-1416

[21] Lord SR, Clark RD, Webster IW. Visual acuity and contrast sensitivity in relation to falls in an elderly population. Age Ageing. 1991;**20**(3):175-181. Available from: https://academic.oup.com/ageing/article-lookup/doi/10.1093/ageing/20.3.175

[22] Lord SR, Menz HB. Visual contributions to postural stability in older adults. Gerontology. 2000;**46**(6): 306-310

[23] Purves D, Augustine GJ, Fitzpatrick D, Hall WC, Lamantia A-S, Mcnamara JO, et al. The Vestibular System. In: Purves D, Augustine GJ, Fitzpatrick D, Hall WC, Lamantia A-S, Mcnamara JO, et al., editors. Neuroscience. 3rd ed. Sunderland: Sinauer Associates; 2004. p. 315–335

[24] Sedó-Cabezón L, Boadas-Vaello P, Soler-Martín C, Llorens J. Vestibular damage in chronic ototoxicity: A mini-review. Neurotoxicology. 2014;**43**:21-27

[25] Tian JR, Shubayev I, Baloh RW, Demer JL. Impairments in the initial horizontal vestibulo-ocular reflex of older humans. Experimental Brain Research. 2001;**137**(3–4):309-322

[26] Gazzola JM, Ganança FF, Aratani MC, Perracini MR, Ganança MM. Clinical evaluation of elderly people with chronic vestibular disorder. Brazilian Journal of Otorhinolaryngology. 2006;**72**(4): 515-522

[27] Grace Gaerlan M, Alpert PT, Cross C, Louis M, Kowalski S. Postural balance in young adults: The role of visual, vestibular and somatosensory systems. Journal of the American Academy of Nurse Practitioners. 2012;**24**(6):375-381

[28] Shaffer SW, Harrison AL. Aging of the somatosensory system: A translational perspective. Physical Therapy. 2007;**87**(2):193-207. Available from: https://academic.oup.com/ptj/ptj/article/2742177/Aging

[29] Lockhart TE, Spaulding JM, Park SH. Age-related slip avoidance strategy while walking over a known slippery floor surface. Gait & Posture. 2007; **26**(1):142-149

[30] Lord S, Ward J. Age-associated differences in sensori-motor function and balance in community dwelling women. Age and Ageing. 1994;**23**(6): 452-460

[31] Turcot K, Sagawa Y, Hoffmeyer P, Suvà D, Armand S. Multi-joint postural behavior in patients with knee osteoarthritis. Knee. 2015;**22**(6):517-521. DOI: 10.1016/j.knee.2014.09.001

[32] Walker CRC, Myles C, Nutton R, Rowe P. Movement of the knee in osteoarthritis. Journal of Bone and Joint Surgery. British Volume. 2001;**83**(2): 195-198

[33] Quintana JM, Arostegui I, Escobar A, Azkarate J, Goenaga JI, Lafuente I. Prevalence of knee and hip osteoarthritis and the appropriateness of joint replacement in an older population. Archives of Internal Medicine. 2008;**168**(14):1576-1584

[34] Barry BK, Carson RG. The consequences of resistance training for movement control in older adults. Journals of Gerontology. Series A, Biological Sciences and Medical Sciences. 2004;**59**(7):730-754. Available from: papers://5a68cd75-9e27-4626-8d94-057f1df96060/Paper/p43

[35] Orr R. Contribution of muscle weakness to postural instability in the elderly. A systematic review. European Journal of Physical and Rehabilitation Medicine. 2010;**46**(2):183-220

[36] Persad C, Cook S, Giordani B. Assessing falls in the elderly: Should we use simple screening tests or a comprehensive fall risk evaluation? European Journal of Physical and Rehabilitation Medicine. 2010;**46**(2): 249-259

[37] Hatton AL, Rome K, Dixon J, Martin DJ, McKeon PO. Footwear interventions: A review of their sensorimotor and mechanical effects on balance performance and gait in older adults. Journal of the American Podiatric Medical Association. 2013; **103**(6):516-533. Available from: http://www.ncbi.nlm.nih.gov/pubmed/24297988

[38] Springer BA, Marin R, Cyhan T, Roberts H, Gill NW. Normative values for the unipedal stance test with eyes open and closed. Journal of Geriatric Physical Therapy [Internet]. 2007;**30**(1):8-15. Available from: http://www.ncbi.nlm.nih.gov/pubmed/19839175

[39] de Waroquier-Leroy L, Bleuse S, Serafi R, Watelain E, Pardessus V, Tiffreau AV, et al. The Functional Reach Test: Strategies, performance and the influence of age. Annals of Physical and Rehabilitation Medicine. 2014; **57**(6):452-464. DOI: 10.1016/j.rehab.2014.03.003

[40] Duncan PW, Weiner DK, Chandler J, Studenski S. Functional reach: A new clinical measure of balance. Journals of Gerontology. 1990;**45**(6):M192-M197. Available from: https://academic.oup.com/geronj/article-lookup/doi/10.1093/geronj/45.6.M192

[41] Cesari M, Kritchevsky SB, Penninx BWHJ, Nicklas BJ, Simonsick EM, Newman AB, et al. Prognostic value of usual gait speed in well-functioning older people—Results from the health, aging and body composition study. Journal of the American Geriatrics Society. 2005; **53**(10):1675-1680

[42] Studenski S, Perera S, Wallace D, Chandler JM, Duncan PW, Rooney E, et al. Physical performance measures in the clinical setting. Journal of the American Geriatrics Society. 2003; **51**(3):314-322. Available from: http://www.ncbi.nlm.nih.gov/pubmed/12588574

[43] Graham J, Ostir G. Assessing walking speed in clinical research: A systematic review. Journal of Evaluation in Clinical Practice. 2008;**14**(4):552-562. Available from: http://onlinelibrary.wiley.com/doi/10.1111/j.1365-2753.2007.00917.x/full

[44] Graham JE, Ostir GV, Kuo YF, Fisher SR, Ottenbacher KJ. Relationship between test methodology and mean velocity in timed walk tests: A review. Archives of Physical Medicine and Rehabilitation. 2008;**89**(5):865-872

[45] Berg K. Measuring balance in the elderly: Preliminary development of an instrument. Physiotherapy Canada. 1989;**41**(6):304-311. Available from: https://utpjournals.press/doi/10.3138/ptc.41.6.304

[46] Santos GM, Souza ACS, Virtuoso JF, Tavares GMS, Mazo GZ. Valores preditivos para o risco de queda em idosos praticantes e não praticantes de atividade física por meio do uso da escala de equilíbrio de berg. Revista Brasileira de Fisioterapia. 2011;**15**(2): 95-101

[47] Guralnik JM, Simonsick EM, Ferrucci L, Glynn RJ, Berkman LF, Blazer DG, et al. A short physical performance battery assessing lower extremity function: Association with self-reported disability and prediction of mortality and nursing home admission. Journals of Gerontology. 1994;**49**(2):M85-M94. Available from: https://academic.oup.com/geronj/article-lookup/doi/10.1093/geronj/49.2.M85

[48] Veronese N, Bolzetta F, Toffanello ED, Zambon S, De Rui M, Perissinotto E, et al. Association between short physical performance battery and falls in older people: The Progetto Veneto Anziani Study. Rejuvenation Research. 2014;**17**(3):276-284. Available from: http://online.liebertpub.com/doi/abs/10.1089/rej.2013.1491

[49] Podsiadlo D, Richadson S. The timed "Up and Go" test: A test of basic functional mobility for frail elderly persons. Journal of the American Geriatrics Society. 1991;**39**(2): 142-148

[50] Rose D, Jones C, Lucchese N. Predicting the probability of falls in community-residing older adults using the 8-foot up- and-go: A new measure of functional mobility. Journal of Aging and Physical Activity. 2002;**10**(4): 466-475

[51] Costa J, Gonçalves C, Rodrigues G, de Paula A, Pereira M, Safons M. Exercícios multisensoriais no equilíbrio e na prevenção de quedas em idosos [Internet]. 2009. Available from: http://www.efdeportes.com/efd135/exercicios-multisensoriais-em-idosos.htm

[52] Prata MG, Scheicher ME. Effects of strength and balance training on the mobility, fear of falling and grip strength of elderly female fallers, Journal of Bodywork and Movement Therapies. 2015;**19**(4):646-650. DOI: 10.1016/j.jbmt.2014.11.013

[53] Gil-Gómez JA, Lloréns R, Alcñiz M, Colomer C. Effectiveness of a Wii balance board-based system (eBaViR) for balance rehabilitation: A pilot randomized clinical trial in patients with acquired brain injury. Journal of NeuroEngineering and Rehabilitation. 2011;**8**(1):30 Available from: http://www.jneuroengrehab.com/content/8/1/30

[54] Clark RA, Bryant AL, Pua Y, McCrory P, Bennell K, Hunt M. Validity and reliability of the Nintendo Wii Balance Board for assessment of standing balance. Gait Posture. 2010; **31**(3):307-310. Available from: https://www.sciencedirect.com/science/article/pii/S096663620900664X?via%3Dihub

[55] Carvalho IF, Leme GLM, Scheicher ME. The influence of video game training with and without subpatelar bandage in mobility and gait speed on elderly female fallers. Journal of Aging Research [Internet]. 2018;**2018**: 9415093. Published 2018 Mar 26. DOI: 10.1155/2018/9415093

[56] Visintin M, Barbeau H. The effects of body weight support on the locomotor pattern of spastic paretic patients. Canadian Journal of Neurological Sciences. 1989;**16**(3): 315-325

[57] Dietz V. Spinal cord pattern generators for locomotion. Clinical Neurophysiology. 2003;**114**(8): 1379-1389

[58] Asanuma H, Keller A. Neuronal mechanisms of motor learning in mammals. Neuroreport. 1991;**2**:217-224

[59] Toole T, Maitland C, Warren E, Hubmann M, Panton L. The effects of loading and unloading treadmill walking on balance, gait, fall risk, and daily function in Parkinsonism. NeuroRehabilitation. 2005;**20**(4): 302-322

[60] Frenkel-Toledo S, Giladi N, Peretz C, Herman T, Gruendlinger L, Hausdorff JM. Treadmill walking as an external pacemaker to improve gait rhythm and stability in Parkinson's disease. Movement Disorders. 2005; **20**(9):1109-1114

[61] Herman T, Giladi N, Gruendlinger L, Hausdorff JM. Six weeks of intensive treadmill training improves gait and quality of life in patients with Parkinson's disease: A pilot study. Archives of Physical Medicine and Rehabilitation. 2007;**88**(9):1154-1158

[62] Abbasian S, Rastegar MMM. Is the intensity or duration of treadmill training important for stroke patients? A meta-analysis. Journal of Stroke & Cerebrovascular Diseases. 2018; **27**(1):32-43. DOI: 10.1016/j. jstrokecerebrovasdis.2017.09.061

[63] Sullivan KJ, Brown DA, Klassen T, Mulroy S, Ge T, Azen SP, et al. Effects of task-specific locomotor and strength training in adults who were ambulatory after stroke: Results of the STEPS randomized clinical trial. Physical Therapy. 2007;**87**(12):1580-1602. Available from: https://academic.oup.com/ptj/article-lookup/doi/10.2522/ptj.20060310

[64] Barbeau H, Visintin M. Optimal outcomes obtained with body-weight support combined with treadmill training in stroke subjects. Archives of Physical Medicine and Rehabilitation. 2003;**84**(10):1458-1465

[65] Hesse S. Treadmill training with partial body weight support after stroke: A review. NeuroRehabilitation. 2008; **23**(1):55-65

[66] Bjornson KF, Moreau N, Bodkin AW. Short-burst interval treadmill training walking capacity and performance in cerebral palsy: A pilot study. Developmental Neurorehabilitation. 2018;**16**:1-8. Available from: https://www.tandfonline.com/doi/full/10.1080/17518423.2018.1462270

[67] Mattern-Baxter K, McNeil S, Mansoor JK. Effects of home-based locomotor treadmill training on Gross Motor Function in young children with cerebral palsy: A quasi-randomized controlled trial. Archives of Physical Medicine and Rehabilitation. 2013;**94**(11):2061-2067. DOI: 10.1016/j. apmr.2013.05.012

[68] Dorfman M, Herman T, Brozgol M, Shema S, Weiss A, Hausdorff J, et al. Dual-task training on a treadmill to improve gait and cognitive function in elderly idiopathic fallers. Journal of Neurologic Physical Therapy. 2014; **38**(4):246-253

[69] van Ooijen MW, Roerdink M, Trekop M, Visschedijk J, Janssen TW, Beek PJ. Functional gait rehabilitation in elderly people following a fall-related hip fracture using a treadmill with visual context: Design of a randomized controlled trial. BMC Geriatrics. 2013; **13**:34